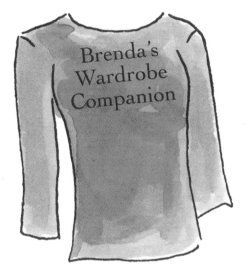

Brenda's
Wardrobe
Companion

Also by Brenda Kinsel

40 over 40:
40 Things Every Woman Over 40
Needs to Know About Getting Dressed

In the Dressing Room with Brenda:
A Fun and Practical Guide
to Buying Smart and Looking Great

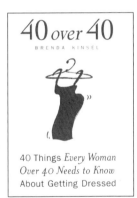

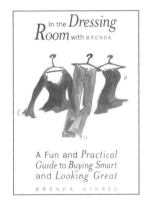

Brenda's Wardrobe Companion

A Guide to Getting Dressed from the Inside Out

BY BRENDA KINSEL

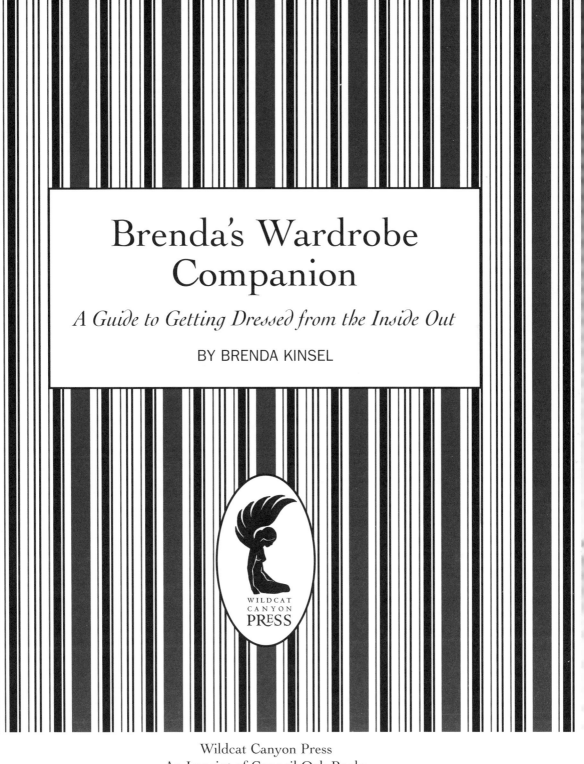

WILDCAT
CANYON
PRESS

Wildcat Canyon Press
An Imprint of Council Oak Books
San Francisco / Tulsa

Cover design and interior art direction:
Jenny M. Phillips of JuMP Studio
Interior layout:
Shannon Laskey
Typographic Specifications:
Body text set in Cochin, additional text set in Franklin Gothic, Handwriting and Nobel

Printed in Canada
Library of Congress Cataloging-in-Publication Data
Kinsel, Brenda, 1952-
Brenda's wardrobe companion/
by Brenda Kinsel.
p. cm.
ISBN 1-885171-71-4
1. Clothing and dress-Handbooks, manuals, etc.
2. Fashion-Handbooks, manuals, etc. I. Title.
TT507 .K563 2002
646'.34—dc21
2002012199

03 04 05 06 07 5 4 3 2 1

Contents

Dedication

To my buddy forever, Patricia Clure, with love.

Acknowledgements, Hugs and Kisses

An unbelievable force stands behind every book that reaches a store shelf. Having now experienced this personally three times, I appreciate it with deep reverence. Let me share some of the force that has been behind this book.

I want to thank Tamara Traeder and Patsy Barich of Wildcat Canyon Press and Paulette Millichap and Ja-lene Clark of Council Oak Books for their passion and commitment to women and women's issues. Thank you for standing behind this project and helping to send it out into the world.

Thank you, Jenny Phillips, for your brilliance in creating the energy and beauty through your illustrations and book design that drives these words right off the page and into the minds and hearts of readers. Thanks to Shannon Laskey for all the great ideas in layout. This project was especially complicated by all the different elements and yet you both made every page a delight to look at. Thank you!

Thank you to the people who provided extra expertise to sections of this book: Persia Matine (hair and makeup tips), Toni Bernbaum (collage ideas), Erin Kinsel (style glossary) and Helena Chenn (fit expertise).

Thank you to Toni Bernbaum (again), who came in at the end of the project for a "quick read" that lasted two weeks. Through floods, power outages, and Christmas, she sat in my office with me polishing this book. Thank you to Ja-lene Clark who also came in full force in the last weeks of the project and held the light for all to see so the technical work could be completed skillfully. Your perseverance and commitment are awesome.

Creating a manuscript takes a few key ingredients: paper, coffee, music, and understanding friends and family members who don't take the words "I just need to be alone!!!!" personally. The most difficult thing to do is to get one's butt into the seat of the chair that faces the computer. Christie Nelson, my writing buddy, is the kind person who can push me like a gale force wind into that chair. Thank you so much for your endless encouragement, suggestions, compassion and commitment to me and the women reading this book.

Because it would be easy to sit in one's studio and do crossword puzzles rather than write a book (because no one knows what you're doing out there anyway), I must acknowledge the people responsible for the moral and spiritual support that is needed to get through a big project like this. Thank you to my blessed 7 @ 7 group (Nadine, Joan, Joanne, Christa, Kate and Rosemary), the Connections group and our mighty leader, Gayle Swift.

Thanks to Randi Merzon and Linda Anderson for your loving support particularly in showing me the beauty of writing in a way that is sustainable while reminding me of the importance of balance in my life. Thank you to my parents, Don and Alma Reiten, whose finest parenting is making my years golden.

To Pattiricia (Patti + Patricia = Pattiricia) Clure, so many thanks. You are my rock. Thank you for championing my left-hand writing voice. With loving wisdom, you always help me make sense of my precious life. Thank you for your listening ear and your steady love. Immeasurable love and appreciation to two more rocks, Louise Elerding and Kim Connor Kuhn.

Thank you to the Bella Group — Huda Baak, Lynn Sydney and Marjory DeRoeck. Your vision is priceless.

Big loving hugs to my best friends in Fargo, North Dakota, Jack Sunday and Sandy Buttweiler of the Jack and Sandy Show on KFGO radio. Our bi-monthly shows keep me feeling frisky. Thanks so much! I love you guys!

To my precious Russ Gelardi who completely blew to smithereens the notion of meeting my deadlines using the white knuckle, isolated, tortured, hair-pulling technique. Your sweet love, kindness, faith, and patience flowed generously and kept me a happy writer. Thank you from every inch of my heart.

To my great kids who make life so rich for me: Caity, Erin, and Trevor. You bring me such pleasure, courage and love. Thank you.

And to those people who have been my guiding force for these last almost twenty years, my clients. Your truth, stories, and brilliance inspire me constantly. Much, much love.

Editorial Note
Some individuals' names have been changed and certain characteristics have been disguised to protect contributors' privacy.

Introduction

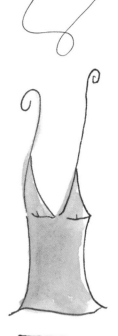

Nearly twenty years ago, while I was deciding on my career, I had one of those bolt-of-lightning moments. I asked myself, Is this attention to fashion, beauty, and looking good worthwhile when there are diseases to be cured, illiteracy to be fought, the poor to be fed and housed? How does this fit with my spiritual values? I didn't have the answer.

For nine months I kept quiet. Not one peep about colors, fabrics, silhouettes, fashion trends, lipstick colors, hairstyles. Not a word. One day I was visiting a cousin of mine. She had a friend over who was getting into the workplace after years of staying at home. "Home" for her was a rural community where she kept goats and chickens and where her dress code was jeans and her husband's worn plaid shirt. She was going to be commuting to the city, working with other professionals who'd been with the company for years. She'd be putting on heels, pantyhose, skirts, jackets, and blouses. (It was the 1980s, before casual dress codes had been introduced.)

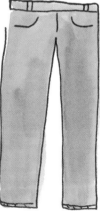

She was as nervous as a cow in a thunderstorm. She wanted to fit in — right away. **She wanted to look the part so she could do the part.** There was enough pressure in her job; she didn't need to worry about what other people would think if she showed up looking like she was just off the farm. She felt anxious and didn't know where to turn. She was lost.

In spite of my locked-jaw vow to keep silent about clothes, I couldn't help myself. My mouth opened and out spilled all these ideas: which colors would give her authority, what fabrics to look for in suits, what accessories she could add that would add to her credibility. By outfitting her, I replaced her doubts with confidence. I erased her insecurity which allowed her to experience ease. Together we transformed the problems so she could go out there and do a good job, gain the confidence of her peers, and bring home a paycheck that would help her family. I was taking away the biggest obstacle she had so she could do what she knew how to do — her job.

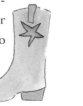

The expression in her eyes turned from worry to excitement. Her mood changed from being heavy to exuberant. The glitches were gone. *She was free.*

I left, got in my car, and drove down San Anselmo Avenue, passing the shops and delis, thinking about what had just happened. Oh my gosh, I thought. What could I have done that would have been more spiritually satisfying than helping this woman just now?

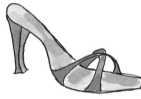

In that second, my nine-month hiatus was over. I was determined to help others achieve their goals by making their clothes a non-issue. I was convinced that helping women look their best and feel comfortable with themselves was definitely a worthwhile career choice.

Nearly twenty years have passed since then. What I've noticed is every woman asks questions like these: Is it vain to think about clothes? Is it frivolous to spend time putting outfits together? If I get attention for my looks, will people not notice my brain? As long as there are homeless people, how can I be so selfish? If I suddenly look great, won't my friends hate me or think I'm full of myself?

If you're holding back from expressing your true wonderful self effortlessly in clothes, what are the reasons why? It takes too much time? Too much money? You don't want people to think you focus on your appearance? You want to be valued for other things? Have I hit on any of your concerns yet?

IF NOT, TELL ME YOUR CONCERNS RIGHT NOW:

If I look great, then _____

If I spend money on myself, then _____

If I spend time on myself, then _____

Here's the catch. If you're a success at being invisible or not standing out, it's going to take a long time to get noticed for the things you do want to be known for.

Here's the thing. Clothes — colors, shapes, patterns — are all tools to bring out whatever you want to bring out. It's your choice. Want to emphasize how approachable you are? Wear medium-toned colors in soft fabrics. Want to get noticed for your efficiency? Avoid jangly jewelry. Leave your Mickey Mouse watch at home and wear your stainless steel one. Get noticed for what you want to be noticed for and use clothes to do it.

TOP 10 REASONS FOR FOCUSING ON YOURSELF AND CLOTHES:

1. Learning who you are is a lifelong spiritual process. Dressing the person you are helps you see yourself.

2. Your being your beautiful and natural self is an inspiration to your family and others.

3. Dressing is your opportunity to be creative every day.

4. Beauty is healing. It's nurturing and nourishing. Don't deny your beauty.

5. Clothes help you get noticed for the right reasons. Choosing to express yourself in clothes is both wonderful and powerful.

6. Clothes are an investment in yourself. Invest wisely by using your money to buy the right things only after you've taken the time to learn what those right things are.

7. The physical body is a beautiful thing. Adorning it is a way to honor the body.

8. Dressing well frees you to forget about your clothes and concentrate on living.

9. Dressing carefully and lovingly shows you respect yourself.

10. When you take care of yourself—your clothes and your grooming—it gives others confidence that you do the same in your personal and professional affairs.

Why not get noticed for what you WANT to get noticed for?

How do I know this? Because I have witnessed it for nearly two decades through my business, Inside Out, A Style and Wardrobe Consulting Company. All the women I have worked with, from San Francisco to Stockholm, have learned through my program of getting dressed from the inside out, that by learning about themselves and clothes, they experience more pleasure, confidence, and happiness than they ever thought they could. I want you to have what they have. Through this book I've brought you all my years of experience working with women of every age and size. Exercises I do with them, I will do with you in these pages. The tips I give them in the dressing room, I share with you here. Everything I do with them, I do with you and more! I believe it is the right of every woman to express herself joyfully and effortlessly in clothes. I want you to enjoy that right. I'll teach you how. Now join me.

Have I convinced you yet? Don't neglect yourself one more second. Don't forget who you are and what you want. Get dressed and remind yourself. You're alive! You're here! You are making a contribution! It makes sense to let clothes help you do that because that's exactly what they love to do. Don't let some excuse hold you back from experiencing the

joy in the simple act of getting dressed.

How to Use This Book

GREETINGS, DEAR READER! Having picked up this book and looked at the intro, I expect you're now paging through and wondering: Is there really something here that'll grab me, shake me up, turn me around? Well, I'm here to tell you — yes! There is! Plenty! *You're going to learn that by changing your clothes, you will change your life* — in goosebump kinds of ways. The right clothes on your body are going to make you excited about getting up in the morning and thrilled to be going out at night. Life is going to look a lot rosier. And let me tell you, rosy looks good on you.

But hey, we've only just met. You have a right to be skeptical. "Come on, Brenda," you're saying. "If I change my clothes, my life will change? My life and clothes aren't half bad. Maybe I don't need any help." **How about taking this little test?** See how you do on the Fashion Quiz on page seven and then we'll discuss whether we could improve things or not.

⟶

Okay, how'd you do? If you're like most women, you've answered yes to many, maybe even most, of these questions. What is it about clothes that keeps us stumbling even though we're smart, accomplished, and generally very capable people? We're going about it all wrong, that's what. We take advice from people who know less than we do about what's right for us, but because they have an authoritative tone, we listen to them. We read magazines that propose solutions to our problems, but we can't quite apply the answers to our situations. We feel guilty about focusing attention on our looks when there are so many more important things to attend to. Believe me, there are dozens of reasons why, after all these years of putting clothes on our bodies, we still aren't getting it right.

FASHION QUIZ:
Answer YES or NO to the following lucky 13 questions:

1. Do you put off taking care of your clothing needs until you lose weight, you win the lottery, the divorce becomes final, or the kids grow up?

2. Do you pay attention only to clothes you wear out in public and wear clothes at home that you wouldn't otherwise be caught dead in?

3. Do you open your closet door and find nothing to wear even though your closet is stuffed to overflowing?

4. Does the word "accessories" fill you with terror, dread, feelings of inadequacy or conjure up dated images of tiaras, boas, and kid gloves?

5. Are you typically late for work or parties because it takes you forever to figure out what to wear?

6. Do you pack for a trip and lug around suitcases full of clothes you never wear?

7. When you receive a compliment on how you look, do you feel confused about exactly what you did to earn that compliment?

8. Do you have clothes in your closet that you never wear—like lime-green bridesmaids' dresses with pumps to match, maternity tops with ruffled collars, anything size 6, souvenir clothes you picked up in Guatemala, China, Hawaii, Florida?

9. Are you mistaken for the secretary when you're head of the firm, or for the grandmother when you're the mother? Do people treat you like you're less together than you really are?

10. Do you avoid shopping because you're intimidated by salespeople?

11. Do you believe that a sense of style belongs only to a select few and you're not one of them?

12. Do you go shopping with friends or family (spouse, mother, your children) and come home with what they like, not necessarily what you like?

13. Do you dress out of obligation without ever enjoying the feel of a fabric, loving the color of something, or experiencing a sense of well-being in your clothes?

But here's the good news. Armed with new information, your relationship to clothes will be changed forever. Rather than being at the mercy of an aggressive salesperson, the latest fashion trend, or a big sister who thinks she knows what's best for you, you are going to be the commander of your clothes destiny. With restored faith in yourself and your decision-making abilities, you'll be thrilled with your wardrobe! How about that? Sounds great, doesn't it?

Okay, you've got some things to learn. You have some principles to adopt, some homework to do. You're not going to have this handled by noon tomorrow, but it is a very do-able project. I've created endless amounts of support for you so you'll be wildly successful. *Trust me.*

The first thing you need for that wildly successful relationship with clothes is to believe you have it coming. I've heard every reason imaginable why women think they can't have a great relationship with their wardrobes. Well, maybe not every reason. Maybe you'll have one I haven't heard of yet. It doesn't matter. You can bring me bushels and bushels of reasons why you can't have what you want, and I will bring in semi-truckloads of reasons why you can.

Give Me Liberty!

There are certain things that I want every woman to expect from herself and her clothes. Let's call them wardrobe liberties. My hope is you believe you are entitled to them, too. Because when you do, you and your clothes get along and are happy.

The problem is, some women believe that things just don't work out. They believe they'll never have an easy time with clothes no matter what. If this is you, I want to turn your head around. If you're feeling hopeless about clothes, there is hope!

I have written the Wardrobe Bill of Rights, and I'd like you to tear this page out and tack it up in your closet. Photocopy it and pass it around to all your friends. Fold up a copy and keep it in your wallet or your glove compartment. Read it repeatedly. Believe it, embrace it, celebrate it. Let this Wardrobe Bill of Rights liberate you from all those reasons why you can't look and feel fabulous in your clothes. Before you experience ease and delight in everything you put on your body, you need to accept your right to have it be so.

Read through the following and then do me a favor. Sign it and date it. I'm serious. Commit to these principles. You don't have to know the "how" part yet. That's coming. Just take this first step in agreeing to your right to have this in your life. Don't squirm. Be bold. Read and sign.

THE WARDROBE BILL OF RIGHTS

1. I have the right to open my closet door and have everything I see work for me 100 percent—to be the right colors, fit perfectly, feel great, and look great on me.

2. I have the right to buy only what I love and not settle for kinda, sorta, close, maybe, or "it'll do."

3. I have the right to take all the time I need and get all the information I need to really understand what works best on my body.

4. I have the right to know what I really like and to be adorned every day by those things.

5. I have the right to focus on my needs and have them met.

6. I have the right to spend money on myself.

7. I have the right to get help in this area without feeling like I've failed or that I'm inadequate or deficient in some way.

8. I have the right to please myself with my choice of everything I wear from my underwear to my socks to the umbrella I use in the rain.

9. I have the right to have this part of my life run smoothly so I can get on with all the other things that are important to me.

10. I have the right to total ease and pleasure in getting dressed.

SIGNED_____ DATE _____

Welcome! You are at the threshold of a new and vastly improved experience with clothes. I might as well tell you now — this book is about a whole lot more than clothes and what looks good with what. This workbook serves as a guide to expressing yourself as effortlessly as a rose expresses its radiance in a summer garden. I'm not being flip here. I am dead serious. I love clothes. I love the art of dressing well. I love seeing a woman on the street who really has it going on: well-groomed, looking sharp, confident, and put together. But more importantly, it's how well clothes match a woman's essence and support her in what she's up to in life that's my pure delight. And that's what I'll show you how to do. I'll show you how to be that put-together woman — distinguished in a way that suits you perfectly, whether that's in a quiet understated way, a playful artistic way, a reserved and proper way, or a dramatic, over-the-top way — YOUR way!

By changing your clothes to the ones that enhance, emphasize and flatter, you become a better version of yourself.

Change Your Clothes, Change Your Life

Some clothes have a nasty habit of disguising, hiding, diminishing, and undervaluing you. In the right clothes, you can see both your inner and outer beauty, and so can others. You can see the truth about yourself and reflect that truth every day. Come meet a few people who by changing their clothes, changed their lives.

CAROL had neglected her wardrobe and her image for years. We worked in her closet and did some shopping together, updating her style and bringing out a "quietly powerful" look through her clothes. She demonstrated through her put-together look that she respected and honored herself. That's when a long-standing strained relationship she had with abusive family members began to change. These same people responded to her new look by treating her with more consideration and respect.

KAREN grew up very neglected around clothes. She was poorly dressed, always cold, and had holes in her shoes. She was put down by her family for wanting the things other girls had. As an adult, she didn't have a clue how to shop for herself. She wept for joy on our first shopping trip when she saw how beautiful she looked in the right choices for her. She embraced her right to express who she was. Learning how to dress herself with care is one of the most important things she's ever done for herself. She says, "It's like a parenting process, a developmental process that I'd never experienced." Her new knowledge about clothes gave her self-confidence, self-esteem, and an emotional well-being that she'd never known.

You'll meet more women and hear their stories as you read along. I want you to know that what happened to them can happen to you too! They went through the same steps you're about to take.

Here's Why

When you dress like someone other than who you are, you're not inhabiting yourself as you really are. If you throw just anything on, you aren't focused. You miss meeting the right people. Opportunities may not notice you.

You are a gem. And just as gems with clarity are more valuable, you with clarity are more valuable to yourself and to others. The best-chosen clothes for you will clarify and polish who you are.

In order to find your look in clothes, let's dig deep into your psyche first. Things will emerge that will surprise, amuse, and delight you. This workbook will help you discover who you are and I'll show you how to express that through clothes.

You express your individuality in many ways already — in how you put a home together, in the handwritten notes you send to loved ones, in the way you assemble family photo albums, entertain friends, tend your garden, cook your meals. Now you're going to put your personal stamp on how you present yourself by the way you wear clothes.

Oh yes, you'll learn how to accentuate your assets, how to wear colors that flatter you, **how to shop,** and so much more. In this workbook, I give you a step-by-step process that teaches you to really honor yourself. It's my experience that women are famous for neglecting themselves in subtle, habitual ways. The care-giving qualities that we are famous for are wonderful, but they also entice us to invest our energy in others while leaving ourselves bankrupt. Jobs, husbands, family, community commitments all vie for top billing in our lives. How many stories have you heard like this one? A friend loses a loved one and she shares, "Wow, we are just here for a wink. What am I waiting for? I want to experience more joy in my life!"

Panic is a great motivator. Receive an invitation to a college reunion and you've got a pressing reason to march into a dressing room, especially if your wardrobe expired two decades ago. Physical changes, like weight gains or losses where nothing fits anymore, will quicken your step to the shopping mall. When there's someone important to impress like a potential boss or a mother-in-law and making the right first impression can be pivotal, knowledge about what looks most flattering to you is suddenly a top priority. When you are in life situations that make you squirm, looking at a wardrobe that's deficient is really depressing.

Maybe you reached for this book without a fire under you. That's great. You're the one I'm prepared to work even harder for. It's easy to fall into a rut and get sleepy around your clothes just like people get sleepy in a marriage or a job. A wardrobe that's been around a long time can be dull and boring. I'm here to tell you that a wardrobe that is less than fulfilling, less than enticing, exciting, or meaningful is just not good enough for you or your friends. **I want to raise the standards you live by.** I want to rattle your wardrobe cage.

Let's Make a Deal

I'll supply you with style and wardrobe solutions where your clothes act like your best friends. They'll be supportive, encouraging, happy to see you, and eager to show you a good time. I'll share stories of inspiration and transformation that have come from nearly twenty years of working with women and their clothes. I'll bring everything I know into this workbook to make it as intimate, real, and rewarding to you as possible.

Here's what I ask in return. **I want your honesty.** I want you to tell me (and maybe a buddy, but more about that later) the truth about your dreams, desires, hopes, needs, and wants. I want the truth about what you think stands in the way of your having those things in your life. I want you to be willing to dig down to the deepest truths about yourself and bring me that raw material.

You may resist. You may think you don't want me to see the gritty stuff. That's okay. Trust me. I can handle the disappointment, bitterness, resistance, defeat, and complaints that live inside you. I know what to do with it.

What I often find is there's a lot of pain that has to break up and get out of the way before you can dress yourself with joy. I'll trade you your pain and insecurities and give you what you deserve — your true and beautiful natural self. Mom's disappointment about your never wearing the frilly dresses she wanted you to is exactly what I'm looking for. The terror of switching from a school where kids wore uniforms to a public school where kids wore anything could be the stumbling block we examine before you move on to confidence with clothes. Becoming aware of the comparisons to your older (or, perhaps, younger) sister is the perfect passage for finding freedom now and dressing yourself with pleasure. Let's roll up our sleeves and get in there.

Stay with me through the exercises in this book, and you'll *free yourself* from restrictions that were created years ago and have no place in your current life. We heal. **Clothes can help.** They can be the salve that brings love and delight to your life. Clothes refresh, rejuvenate, and renew.

What is it about clothes that keeps us stumbling even though we're smart, accomplished, and generally very capable people?

Tell the Truth

You will gain the most from this book by expressing your truth. I'm going to give exercises to help access that truth. What I want you to do is just let it all spill out.

Here's why. When you tell the truth, almost magically, grace comes forward to support you. I'm not talking out of my nostrils here. It's happened to you. It's happened to me. It happened to Sandra.

SANDRA was in a live-in relationship with a man who was, frankly, boring. While she'd brought him home to meet her parents and they'd even discussed marriage, one day she just sat down and told herself the truth. He was not the man she wanted to be with forever. It wasn't satisfying and she didn't believe that time could change the relationship significantly. Over dinner that night she told him how she felt. Once she heard herself tell the truth, she knew it was over and she had to leave. The phone rang and it was a co-worker. Sandra told her co-worker what had transpired and her co-worker said, "I have an extra bedroom. Why don't you come and stay here until you figure out where you want to be?" In twenty-four hours, Sandra had moved out and on with her life. Once she told the truth, she was no longer stuck. It was as if the valet attendant brought her car around so she could get in and move on.

We've all done it — told the truth and grace supplied the flying carpet that took us to a better place. When you tell the truth in this book, **clothes can be part of that magic carpet ride that gets you where you need to go.**

The Kim Story

When I met KIM twelve years ago, she was working as a pharmacist, as her father and brother had before her. Her hobby was flower arranging. She took classes in that on weekends.

Before each new fashion season, I always ask my clients (and I'll be asking you), "Is there something new in you that wants to be expressed? Have you made some changes that we need to consider?" When I asked Kim this question a few years back, she told me that she was tired of being a health-care provider. She didn't want to be seen as an on-call comforting person 24/7. Now, Kim's kindness is one of the jewels in her crown. No one can miss it once they've met her.

But something else wanted to be expressed. I asked her more about that part. She told me she was really interested in flowers and had even entertained the thought of leaving pharmacy and maybe, MAYBE one day becoming a florist. The thought was so scary to her she almost didn't tell me about it. I knew we had to change her clothes first. She needed to see herself express this arty part in order to gain support in the new direction she was heading.

Kim, petite and adorable, was tired of the nice girl role. In her personal life, she wanted to be more edgy. She didn't want people to take her for granted. She needed more strength and presence in her appearance. She wanted a vacation from people's problems. So that year we created roadblocks and detours so people wouldn't assume they could constantly tell her their troubles. Rather than dressing her in warm soft colors — peach and lilac — I dressed her in black to create an edge. Against the black we mixed in stronger, brighter colors: lime green, bright coral and strong aqua. Instead of floral prints, I dressed her in solids that were more commanding. Instead of soft knits, I put her in clothes that had more body, more crispness. She loved the new look. Her husband loved the new look. She was reminded each day when she got dressed that she was more than a health-care provider. She was a creative, expressive artist and a strong, confident woman.

Kim didn't quit her job right away. She started out by cutting down on her days. For several months she wrestled with the idea of not being a pharmacist. It was a big part of her identity. **Then one day she did it.** She quit the job she'd had for twenty-five years and put her attention on floral arranging. Within a year she had several accounts. She was creating floral arrangements for large parties and events and meeting all kinds of people in the art field.

The whole time Kim was mentally preparing for this change and even while she was feeling wobbly in this new venture, her clothes led the way, opened doors and added credibility to her new life. **Her wardrobe was the yellow brick road** that took her from her old job to her new career, from dissatisfaction to satisfaction. It's what coaxed her each day to trust herself and follow her dreams.

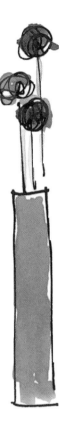

Your Tell-the-Truth-Let-Go-Create Mantra

This program is a process of getting dressed from the inside out. There's a lot of "inside" homework to do before we get to your outsides. The more thoughtfully you do the inside work, the easier it'll be to dress your outsides.

There are three actions you'll be doing over and over again. They are all a part of the wheel that keeps turning and keeping you on track. Remember, as long as you're doing at least one of these actions, you're headed for success.

Tell the truth. I am solely interested in your uncompromised truth telling at every step. I want to know what you love, loathe, desire, and reject. When you tell the truth, you respect yourself.

I spend a lot of time with my clients getting to their truth. Do they like black because they really love it and are crazy about it, or do they have black in their closets because someone said it makes them look thinner? Do they wear a trenchcoat style jacket because they love it, or because it's a hand-me-down from their sister-in-law?

We have the answers inside. We just need to hear ourselves speak them. We know if we love red or teal or pink or orange. We know if we love the feel of cashmere or polished cotton or silk chiffon or corduroy.

We know what nourishes us — whether it's having more energy in our life, which brighter colors would provide, or wearing loose, cuddly clothes made from polar fleece, which we crave for comfort.

So often women accommodate based on what they think they should do. Stop taking care of others. I want to hear what's true for you. Here's your chance to set the record straight. Maybe no one has ever asked you what you thought. *Yippee! Now you have the chance to voice your opinion.* Maybe your thoughts didn't count when you were growing up so you stopped giving them. You provided what was expected of you instead. Being successful in this process is to stand tall, be brave, and tell the truth. Oh boy, are you going to have fun! Telling the truth is like filling the sky full of butterflies. It's beautiful and it's free.

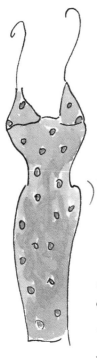

Let go. Once you tell the truth, you discover things in your life that don't match your truth. You love pink but there's no pink in your closet. You love slinky draped clothes but everything you own is stiff and boxy. You love makeup but you never wear it. The next step is letting go of what you've done in the past. When you figure out what you love, it is necessary to let go of everything that doesn't reflect that. Clothes and everything about them are like nutrients. You can't have a healthy wardrobe without the proper nutrients. If the clothes in your closet don't nourish you, let them go and find ones that do. You might have some old, outdated ideas about yourself that have to go as well. You'll be amazed at how good you'll feel when you embrace letting go.

Create. After telling the truth and letting go, you're free to create solutions that bring more happiness. As you let go of the old and the outdated, you open a space where a new vision of yourself can be created based on your truth. In the "creation" phase, anything can happen. Let yourself be surprised by what comes through for you and how the perfect things can show up — like that black, red, blue, and white scarf you spot in a thrift store that's exactly what you want, or an unexpected gift certificate from the new boutique in town that's carrying clothes for your new look.

None of this magic can happen unless you tell the truth, let go, and create.

Find Support from Your History

Remind yourself of all the other times in your life when you told the truth and life shifted giving you a soft landing to fall, no matter what you were going through.

Remembering your past success helps you have the courage to leap again, this time with your clothes and your look. Tell me about the time in your life when you told the truth and it all worked out.

What was the experience?
What was the grace that showed up to help you?

Remember how Sandra was graced by a place to live the very night she broke up with her boyfriend? Expect grace to show up and help you in this project too.

These Are My Expectations of You

I suspect there will be parts of this that are exciting and effortless and parts that will have you feeling like you're walking through mud. It's always easy to start a project, but harder to see it all the way through. It's like going on a diet. Those first few pounds you lose are full of energetic commitment. It's easy. Then the newness wears off, the going gets slower, and you could easily slip back into your old patterns and give up. I'm going to help you push through that. I've created ways for you to feel support at every step.

Here's how this works. There are exercises to do all along the way. Then we work on the outside — putting clothes on you that are just right and organizing your closet so you can enjoy the clothes you've got.

There are lots of writing exercises. Use this workbook to write in your answers or get a special notebook or journal that will capture all the things you're going to discover about yourself. Whichever method you use, decide right now where you're going to keep your materials. It's important to know where your notes are if you aren't keeping them in this book. You'll also be using a three-ring binder, so your notebook, binder (if you use one), and this workbook need to live near each other. I want you to have easy access to the revelations and wise

Buy only what you love and you'll LOVE to use it or wear it!

statements you'll be creating. Decide now: Where will your materials live? In your closet? By your nightstand? In your desk?

HERE'S YOUR NEXT EXERCISE:

"I'm storing my materials _____."

You've made another commitment. Congrats! We're on our way.

Shop for Your Supplies

You need to go out and buy a few things. Start now and use a rule that you'll be reading about again in Attitude Rehab. **BUY ONLY WHAT YOU LOVE.** That's the rule. So when you're buying sheet protectors, think about it. Do you LOVE the matte ones, the glossy ones, the ones with white borders on the edges, or do you want them completely clear? Do you want a white three-ring binder that has a plastic sleeve on the cover into which you can slide pictures? Or maybe you have a favorite color, in which case you might buy a binder in the color you LOVE. Don't be lazy. Don't cut corners. Take time to buy only what you love. Are you with me?

HERE'S WHAT YOU NEED TO GET STARTED:

1. **3-ring binder (2" thick is preferable)**
2. **Plastic sheet protectors**
3. **Dividers**
4. **Glue stick**
5. **Scissors**
6. **Stack of magazines or catalogs**
7. **Notebook or journal that you LOVE and can't wait to write in**
8. **Writing tool that feels great to hold, flows as you write and is a color you LOVE**

Here's the next thing. Make a commitment to time. When do you think you could reasonably get your supplies together? If you put a date down, you are more likely to follow through and get it done. When you let it float, you make a commitment to "whenever."

Set a date instead. This is a support measure to ensure your success. Pick a date that is reasonable and doable.

"I will have my materials collected by _____."

Now that I'm asking you to do things, don't get too carried away about getting it all perfect. I know how it is. We want the right answer now and once we have it, we don't want it to change. However, this is a creative process and creativity by its nature is fluid. How you do this "right now" is perfect for "right now." You'll repeat some of these exercises. The results will be different at different times. So relax. Realize that what you are creating is your masterpiece of the moment. Understand you are in a process that grows and adapts to your changing lifestyle and self-image.

Lighten up and have a good time.

The Buddy System

DO YOU HAVE buddies you call on for help? A friend you walk with at 6 A.M. who shares your enthusiasm for good health? Someone who helps you bake up holiday treats each year? A person you check in with before you make tough decisions? Life runs smoother when your buddies help you through it. When I thought about your going through this step-by-step process — getting dressed from the inside out — I envisioned a buddy being there to help you along the way. So I created a buddy system.

Here's how it works. First, there are many things I'll ask you to do on your own. Then I'll give you a buddy exercise: You'll share information with your buddy, which helps reinforce the new things you are learning about yourself. There are field trips the two of you will go on together, tasks she will do for you in your closet, and just wait until you see how she helps you with decisions in the dressing room! Your buddy is your wardrobe pal. She helps you grow new habits.

8 Things a Buddy Can Do for You

1. Be the voice of reason when you make excuses for a blouse that's too big for you.

2. Hold up your twenty-year-old jeans and give you 12 reasons to dump them. And if it takes 13 reasons, she'll give you 13.

3. Accompany you to the charity where you drop off eight bags of discarded clothes and celebrate with you all the way home.

4. Listen to why you haven't been happy with your clothes and help you identify what's been going wrong.

5. Go with you into the dressing room and help you edit your clothes choices, reminding you that your body is right, it's the clothes that are wrong. She will tirelessly insist that you keep trying things on until you hit the jackpot.

6. Carry the energy bars and water bottles while you shop.

7. Remind you of your shopping plan so you don't end up with ball gowns instead of workout clothes.

8. Pull you out of your ruts when you're heading right for them, like when you're buying yet another long-sleeved black turtleneck.

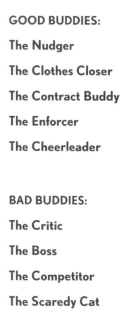

GOOD BUDDIES:

The Nudger

The Clothes Closer

The Contract Buddy

The Enforcer

The Cheerleader

BAD BUDDIES:

The Critic

The Boss

The Competitor

The Scaredy Cat

With the buddy system, you have the opportunity to make a change. It's one thing to have a good hunch about something and another to have that hunch confirmed by someone else. Your buddy will confirm what you already know — that those ratty sweats have got to go.

You're not alone if you find yourself asking, **"Now why couldn't I do that by myself?** Why do I have to have someone else there before I can actually get rid of those sweats when I already know I should?"

Because we get emotionally attached. Having a buddy makes it so much easier to bear the brief moments of grief when we let something go. Plus, it's so much more fun to share the relief when we finally do. Some things are just better done in twos — like paired figure skating, ballroom dancing, and procreating. Some things require a second person. Much of this wardrobe process will benefit from having a second person there to help you.

Me a Buddy, You a Buddy, Be a Buddy Too

There are lots of ways to have and be a buddy. Hopefully you'll have the opportunity to both be one and have one. For now, I'd like you to think about how a buddy can help you. Let me introduce you to a few types of buddies.

The Nudger: I work with clients who are usually well-prepared for our first closet meeting. They have told me over the phone how they have already thrown out six bags of clothes just getting ready for our date. But there's at least 30 percent of their closet that they have doubts about and can't tackle until I'm standing there with them. They need me to give them the final nudge. A buddy can give you a nudge just when you need one.

The clothes closer: Buddies don't need to hover over every step. You might prefer to have a buddy who is a "clothes closer," coming in just at the end of a step, like baseball pitchers who come in fresh at the bottom of the ninth inning to finish things off. Right at the end of your closet clean-out, she could help you take your reject clothes to their next useful place — like a charity, your local thrift store, or your cousin's house. Or she shows up enthusiastically at the end of a shopping trip and helps you make your final decisions. She's a clothes closer.

The contract buddy. You're great at shopping, but you need help when it comes to your closet. Your buddy can come in on a contract basis and help you with specific tasks like arranging your closet for more efficiency, helping you put in shelves, or installing hooks on which to hang your belts.

The enforcer: You can have a buddy who helps you keep your commitments. You may do all of the steps in this process by yourself, but you will have that someone to report to at the end. You can say, "Hey, Marj, I did my homework!" And she can give you a pat on the back — in person, over the phone or by e-mail. It helps to know that someone out there is expecting your call and will celebrate your progress with you.

The cheerleader buddy. Everyone needs a little encouragement from time to time. You may find some steps are as easy to accomplish as finding a seat at the movies on a Tuesday afternoon. Other steps may feel tougher. Your cheerleader buddy can stand behind you, blowing the noisemakers and keeping you energized for each step. She can cheer you on when you finally do the thing you thought you couldn't do — ditch your college wardrobe, complete an outfit head-to-toe, shop for a handbag. She knows when you need a pep talk or a gigglefest that puts a period to your procrastination.

There Are Buddies, and There Are Buddies

Listen carefully to the distinction I am about to make. I am all for having a buddy assist you, but this person has to be someone who will support you. Here are some bad buddy choices.

The critic. This is the person you can't please. She likes the top you pick but tells you it's too expensive to purchase. Or she loves your skirt but tells you it's the wrong length. Nothing satisfies the critic. You're always left with the feeling that nothing you do is right. In this workbook, we are working hard to get rid of the critic in ourselves. It's counterproductive to have a critic for a wardrobe buddy.

The boss. This is the friend you shop with who insists she knows what's best for you. You come home with purchases that stay in your closet for months with the price tags still on. She gets you to take action, but she's not taking the time or doesn't have the sensitivity to really understand you. The boss can keep you from making your own discoveries by jumping in and trying to control things.

The competitor. This is the friend who is always one up on you. If you have a new sweater, she has two in the same style by the end of the week. She secretly strives to stay on top. She's threatened if your changes make you stand out more than she does. The competitor doesn't have your best interests in mind. She wants to be number one and she'll do anything to keep her status. She can't be trusted.

The scaredy cat. Here's a friend who worries about everything you do that's new or different. She's scared of risks and original thought. She's afraid if you move in a new direction without her, she'll lose your friendship. She's invested in your staying small and playing it safe with her. This won't serve you. You need to be able to stretch. Most scaredy cats can't.

Best Buddies

Your buddy needs to be someone who is enthused about clothes or is eager to discover along with you all the things your clothes can do. You might spot good buddy material in someone who always notices when you're wearing a new pair of shoes and is happy for you. Or someone who goes with you to the makeup counter and doesn't let them turn you into a stranger but rather a brighter version of your shining self. Maybe she hears your anxiety at having to attend a function where your

BUDDIES ARE:
Curious
BUDDIES AREN'T:
Know-it-alls

BUDDIES ARE:
Interested in you
BUDDIES AREN'T:
Self-centered

BUDDIES ARE:
Kind
BUDDIES AREN'T:
Pushy

BUDDIES ARE:
Good listeners
BUDDIES AREN'T:
Judgmental

ex-husband's new girlfriend will be and volunteers to help you shop for that killer outfit. Or she possesses skills you don't have. Organizing pantry shelves is her favorite thing while yours is taking the things off the shelves and concocting a splendid soup. Such a buddy would be handy to have when it comes to clearing out your closet, and you'd be invaluable to her when she's putting outfits together in new ways.

If Buddies Aren't Your Bag

Maybe you're a private person and prefer to do things alone. That's fine! There are plenty of ways this workbook will help you make life changes without using a buddy. Where buddy exercises are listed, you can do them with yourself. Make your journal your buddy. Let your binder be your buddy. **Don't forget, I'm your buddy.** Keep my voice in your ear. Take time to process things. You may find that you don't have an official buddy, but you have casual conversations with women friends (inspired by topics you're reading in this book) that creates more support for yourself. Whether you choose to have a buddy or not, you'll get results by learning about the buddy system. You'll learn to be a better buddy to yourself by going inward and listening to your own inner wisdom.

Ask a Buddy

Start thinking about who your buddy might be. Now, start a list of candidates.

MY CANDIDATES:

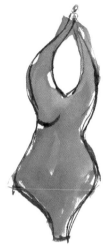

WANTED:
Positive nudger.
Doesn't faint at the
sight of dressing
rooms. Can get
excited about
pleats.

_____

_____

_____

_____

Call them up one at a time. Tell them about this workbook and how the buddy system works. Ask them if they'd like to be your buddy. If more than one says yes, you've created a buddy group. If you all want to do this together, *let the fun begin!* If you do find yourself participating in a buddy group, I suggest you meet once a week. You can rotate houses, thereby getting a chance to see everybody's closet. Plan weekly activities. Set your dates for completing them. Follow this book along and adapt it to your group process. Please let me know how this turns out. I'm serious!

Don't be offended if someone says no. She may be up to her eyeballs in projects and not have time to take on something new right now. Keep trying till you find the person who has the interest, time, and desire to help you out. Remember, you might want to start small. Find a contract buddy to help you with your interview homework and see how it goes.

To the Chosen Buddies Out There

If you've agreed to be someone's buddy, you've been honored. It's your job to be an advocate for your friend. As you help her express more of her true self and her true beauty through her clothes and her appearance, you get the gift of giving.

It is a great service to listen to a friend and take the lead from her. Remember you aren't her. Don't project your personal preferences on her. Listen to her. Work to understand her. You do things for a reason. So does she. **Be curious about her reasons.** Maybe they're valid. Maybe they aren't valid and if you ask good questions, she'll see that they could be replaced with better options. Don't overstep your bounds or make her wrong. You're helping her discover what's right for her. Once she gives you that information, then you're there to help her follow through. And don't worry — in future chapters I'll be giving buddy tips for specific steps. You'll learn how to be a great buddy!

And what's in it for you? The kinder and more generous you are as a buddy, the more likely this wonderfully sensitive person will be a great buddy to you.

The Program

The first step in this program is to have a strong support system in place. Support comes from several sources. Some of it may come

In this workbook, we are working hard to get rid of the critic in ourselves.

from a buddy, if you choose one. Some of it is generated by your own thoughts and self-talk. Some of it comes from your closest friends, family or co-workers who will witness your changes. It's important to get your support system in shape so you can call on it when you need it.

Who Else is Going to Be There for You?

Think about people you know. Who among your friends and family are your strong advocates? It's fair to list people who are no longer living. Did you have a strong advocate in a grandmother who was delighted when she saw you caring for yourself? Put her on the list. Who stands up for you no matter what? Even if you don't choose a buddy, you need support from the people around you.

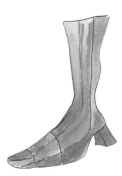

Have a strong support system in place.

MY STRONG ADVOCATES ARE:

_____

_____

_____

_____

_____

Consider also that some people might not be thrilled at the idea of you changing. **Changing your clothes is going to change your life** and not everyone is keen on changes, especially when they feel their lives are impacted — like maybe husbands, best friends, or sisters.

Be discerning. If you end up going out and spending a chunk of money on clothes and come out of the house looking like the most fabulous version of yourself ever, DO NOT walk up to the person who makes you feel the most insecure and say, "What do you think?" She (or he) may respond, "What were you thinking? I liked you the way you used to be. Why did you change?" Just like seedlings need early protection from the elements, wait until the new you has strong roots before you head toward people who could stunt your growth. All opinions are not equal. Don't lay your good news at the doorstep of your biggest critic. Not now. Get used to your new look first.

Who are the sharp-tongued, insecure or tactless people who might want to burst your bubble? List them now and proceed with great caution.

MY CRITICS ARE:

_____

_____

_____

_____

TRY THIS:
Make a collage of people who inspire you. I want you to have strength to draw upon while you are going through this book and doing the exercises. There are so many vulnerable places that come up for women around clothes. It's important to me that you feel supported. Find pictures of people who represent an authenticity that you admire. Choose people who express the qualities you want to express in your life. If they're in your community, ask them for a photo. If they're notable people, cut out their pictures from a magazine or a newspaper. Or they can be people who have passed away. Take a picture of yourself. Put it in the center of a page. Arrange the pictures (or just their names) around yours. Put this page in your binder. Be in good company! These are people whom you admire. Invite them to be on your side. Thank them for being here.

The small voice inside you is saying "You are divine in so many ways!"

What About You?

Even if you choose not to use a buddy, there's a soft, sweet place inside of you that always wants to comfort and support you. I believe that person inside you is just waiting to be your advocate, strength, and courage. I'll help you access that voice in you if it's not already a big part of your life. To get used to this idea, practice accentuating the positive in yourself. *We're going to focus a lot of attention on YOU!* Start coming out of hiding by taking a long, loving look at yourself. I want to hear what makes you unique. How you put your clothes together will be unique too.

Need some nudging? How about the way you decorate your house, the way you care for pets, the way you help friends in need, the way you wrap gifts, the way you make lasagna? Dressing your unique self starts by appreciating your unique self. Go crazy. List a hundred ways you are unique. Use your pretty (and unique) journal if you'd like. Start here.

WHAT'S UNIQUE ABOUT YOU?

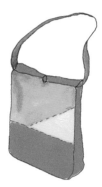

_____

_____

_____

_____

_____

Invite Qualities to Help You

What qualities would be good company for you as you go through this workbook? I can think of a few I'd want — compassion, a sense of fun, understanding, honesty, love, kindness, creativity, joy. Being conscious of these qualities helps you as you learn more about yourself. Just thinking about these words can inspire you.

If you were going to a job interview, it would be a great idea to bring your confidence, clarity, and manners. If you were going to the bedside of a friend, it would be good to bring a bouquet of compassion, love, and hope. So here you are, about to **explore** parts of yourself you haven't explored before. Some hard experiences growing up around clothes might bring up insecurities and past discomfort. What will help you in this exploration? Gather some choice qualities up and have them join you on this project. That's what they are here for.

Don't be shy. Ask for what you want! Tell the truth. You deserve all the help you need. These qualities are ready to show up. Just say their names and they'll be there. List them. Read them often.

QUALITIES:

_____

_____

_____

_____

_____

What are the qualities you want in your suitcase for this part of your journey?

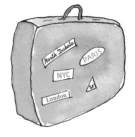

Now here's a simple yet powerful prayer or meditation — whatever you prefer to call it. It's called the Navajo Prayer. You can use any "quality" you like to meditate on. Take "kindness" for example. Here's how it goes:

Kindness before me
Kindness behind me
Kindness to the right of me
Kindness to the left of me
Kindness above me
Kindness below me
Kindness within me
Kindness all around me

Choose a word that inspires you. Put it in this format, and say it out loud. It sets your intention and helps you to see that quality throughout the day. Use it as a tool in the dressing room if you begin to notice that you are being unkind to yourself. It's like cuddling up with a blankey and being comforted by exactly what you need.

When I take walks in the morning near my home, there is a place in the woods where I say the Navajo Prayer. I think of what I especially need that day and whatever word comes to me, I use. Sometimes it's courage, love, guidance, compassion, faith. Try this for a week and track your words. **Does a theme appear?** We all have our strengths and weaknesses. We all have different muscles that need exercise. Let the power of words support you.

JUST FOR FUN:

If you want to see the power of an "inside out" makeover, rent the Bette Davis classic film *Now, Voyager.* Or rent *Working Girl* and watch how Melanie Griffith changed her clothes and went from being the gum-chewing secretary to an authoritative, real player in the business world.

Let Go of What Doesn't Serve Your Progress

Many women carry a lot of useless mental baggage that gets in the way of getting dressed. Things like merciless self-criticism, hopelessness, unrelenting comparisons. Oh gosh, it's ugly. We'll deal with that in the next couple of chapters, but right now just consider what it would be like to free yourself of those bad mental habits. What could you give up now? What could you consider letting go of?

FOR EXAMPLE:

I could give up self-criticism.

I could let go of my hopelessness.

I could give up my comparisons.

I could let go of my self-loathing.

What I want you to know right now is that it's possible to curb those bad habits. Enjoy a cup of tea or some coffee and think about what you are ready to shed. Just like the snake sheds its skin, you can shed some of these scaly things.

FILL IN THE BLANKS:

I'm ready to let go of _____.

I'm ready to give up my _____.

I'm ready to let go of _____.

I'm ready to give up my _____.

BUDDY EXERCISE:
Make a date with your buddy for a little chat over tea, root beer floats or cosmopolitans. Be courageous. Share what you're ready to let go of with your buddy. Chances are she has some of these things on her list too! Explore together what it would be like to have the opposite behavior (hopefulness instead of hopelessness). Ask for her support in letting go of the old and bringing in the new. Let her know the best way she can support you.

Now, let's track how you're doing. If you get through a week or a day or even an hour without criticizing yourself, celebrate. Give yourself a gold star. Write a loving note to yourself and leave it under your pillow. Call your buddy up and **share the good news.** If you have a relapse, then start again. There's no limit to the amount of starts you can take to rid yourself of a bad mental habit.

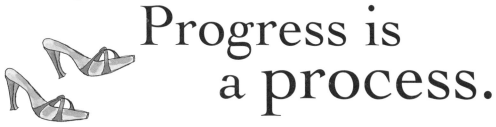 # Progress is a process.

Attitude Rehab:
Breaking Bad Habits

EVERYONE HAS BAD HABITS that have gotten their wardrobes into trouble. And that's just for starters. These habits are also messing with your head. We're going deeper in the next chapter (which may even warrant your having a tissue box nearby). Think of this chapter as the gentle massage and the next one as the deep tissue work. Right now I'm going to give you the easy stuff—premises to live by, starting today, this moment. You don't have to do anything demanding. I'm not asking you to face your closet quagmire or forgive your mother for making you wear that ghastly coat your whole freshman year in high school. You just have to face some nasty habits and be willing to put them to rest from this day forward for as long as you and your buddy both shall live.

Even though some of these fashion strategies that deal with nasty habits may seem like no-brainers, I know from working with my clients, these fashion strategies challenge women from their hair follicles to the polish on their toenails. This could be tough stuff for you too.

Axioms like "do unto others as you would have them do unto you" sound simple, but are hard to practice. It's the same with these. They sound simple, but they threaten your stone-walled belief systems and your compulsive reflexes that are as firmly established as gravity. You may be flabbergasted by one or two of these strategies because you never even realized you had a choice in the matter. But I promise you this—**the freedom and happiness you experience from accepting even one of these new strategies will blow your mind.** And if you embrace every single one as a new guideline, then your life will be completely remodeled and updated. And no, I am not exaggerating. Let's go.

Fashion Strategy #1: Change Your Mind

For every beautiful woman you see walking down the street, there is a woman's voice inside her that rattles off a list of what's "wrong" with her body. The outsides look great, but the insides are polluted with sharp and mean criticisms. "My thighs are too big." "My tummy sticks out." "My upper arms are flabby." "My waist is too thick." "I'm too big-boned." "I've got no butt." "I've got football shoulders."

Magazines sell based on cover stories claiming to solve "problems" women have. The premise is we have problems and we need fixing. Women have problem hair, problem skin, problem relationships. I'll bet you could join in right now with your own list. Stop! I don't want to hear it! All that negative mind chatter makes your life miserable. Changing your clothes is easy. But you're not going to experience true joy in those clothes on your body until you *change your mind*.

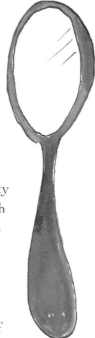

It's hard to find a woman who views her body as a whole. She breaks it into the parts she likes and the parts she hates.

Several years ago I was in a classroom of women studying spiritual work. One thing our teacher repeatedly told us was, "Do not be the first to carve up your own nature." The first time I heard this, it sent shivers through me. I thought about all the times I picked on myself. No one out there was criticizing me. I was the one carving up my own nature.

Do not be the first to carve up your nature. Brutality exists within us. There are cases where the brutality started with an abusive parent, sibling or grandparent. If this happened to you, you can get help to move on. Unfortunately, even after those perpetrators are physically gone from our lives, we continue the pattern—unless we look at it closely and take the necessary steps to heal and let go.

I face this dilemma with my clients. They have all kinds of stories about parts of their bodies they hate. Hate is a strong and over-used word but I've seen women who are delightful and attractive turn the knives on themselves with self-hatred. It's hard to find a woman who views her body as a whole. She breaks it into parts. The parts she likes and the parts she hates. Rarely is the former greater than the latter.

It hurts me to see it and hear it. This is a fierce habit to break, and I beg you to tackle it with me. Do not be the first to carve up your nature. When I can remember that line, the image of carving up my nature is so painful, it stops me cold. I'm hoping it'll stop you too.

Don't alienate your body parts from each other. Your body is a temple that houses your heart and soul. Cherish it all.

CHANGE YOUR MIND:

1. Write out the line, "I will not be the first to carve up my nature." Copy it and put it where you'll see it often.

2. Bodies are tireless miraculous instruments that rarely get the credit they deserve. It's not until something goes wrong — from a hangnail to a broken bone to a disease running wild inside — that we understand and appreciate the value of our bodies. What body parts have you alienated or been disappointed by? Name them. List those parts in the column on the left. Directly across from them, make a list of things that body part does for you.

Body Part   Function/Appreciation

_____   _____

**Give your whole
body a chance
to hear some
thanks from you!**

_____   _____

_____   _____

_____   _____

_____   _____

Indulge yourself. There are ways to be more accepting and kind to the body parts you fret over. Do something wonderful for one of those parts today. Rub your favorite lotion all over those thighs that you criticize. Get a massage and ask the masseur to pay special attention to your upper arms that you find too wiggly. Restore life into that part of your body by bringing loving energy there.

TRY THIS:

Buy something that makes noise and keep it with you in a jacket pocket, your car, or your purse. Yes, I'm serious. You're going to use a noisemaker to startle the nasty thoughts away. When you're in a movie theater watching a scary movie and something really awful comes on the screen, you have the option of covering your eyes and not looking at it, right? When the talk in your mind gets ugly, and degrading things are bouncing around in there, use your noisemaker.

You can interrupt that chatter by making noise. I like those little round toys, round as a quarter and the size of a pot of lip gloss. When you press the center, it makes an animal sound like a bird or a frog. They have them at gift stores that cater to kids. Keep your finger on the center of that thing. Keep repeating that sound until the nasty thoughts stop. Sound is the perfect disrupter. It makes you more conscious of that bad habit when you associate sound with it. Play with this. It works. You'll like it.

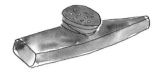

When you feel a "carving" moment coming on, change your mind and appreciate all your body does for you.

Fashion Strategy #2: Focus on What Works

When I work with a woman for the first time, I love making mental notes about all her assets — green eyes, chocolate skin, long legs, striking chestnut brown hair, broad shoulders, pretty hands — and how I want to enhance them. I'm looking at her as though I were looking through a camera lens. To bring her into focus, I pay close attention to her assets and her personality and bring them forward.

At the same time, she's telling me about her problem areas. It's almost compulsive. Women need training to focus on what works. To talk to them about their assets almost seems like a waste of their time. They want me to hurry up and get to the problems.

Hey! The problem is that women aren't focusing on what works! When you focus on what works, those things perceived as challenges become minimized to non-issues. **Who can see the challenges if the assets are being spotlighted?** I want to wave a bright lime-green flag in front of you until you shift your attention from what you think doesn't work to what does work. Hey! Look at your smile, your pretty shoulders, your playful eyes.

It's so common to find women fixated on what they think doesn't work about their bodies. Angeles Arrien, Ph.D., in her book *The Four-Fold Way*, writes about this fixation—calling it an addiction. She says, "When this addiction is fully disengaged, we begin to look at the blessings, gifts, talents, and resources that are available to us in our lives."

I believe that's true, although I might go about approaching it from the opposite way. I suggest that if you honor the blessings, gifts, talents, and resources that are yours, there won't be a place for that fixation to hold onto anymore. The energy it takes to fixate on something is very direct, fierce, and narrow. When you stop fixating on something and open your mind to take in more things, life becomes gentler, more peaceful and more livable. **Fixation isn't fun.** It's limiting and it creates suffering.

I see this in the dressing room all the time. The complaints a woman has about her body disappear when we highlight her assets with her clothing. She experiences more joy and excitement about life without the perceived problem.

Women get fixated on a small part of their physical looks and forget all about the other assets they have—their mental, spiritual, social, and emotional assets. A brilliant woman can fret over the shape of her waist and forget about her riches—her family life, her good work in the world, her devotion to her community. Although this book directs attention to your outsides, it explores your insides as well. We're going to identify all your assets and get them down on paper.

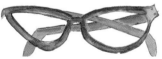

Here's how it works. I'm going to give you an imaginary bank account. Your name is on the account and today you make a deposit so big it'll make your eyes pop. This account is based on your personal value. Not your financial value, but your personal value— your self-worth and self-esteem. Most women start out with bankrupt self-worth. We're going to change all that. I'm giving you a place to deposit and review your assets, like a savings account book or a stock portfolio. I want you to see it in black and white. In this account will go your gifts, talents, blessings, and resources. You'll continue to make deposits in these accounts as time goes on. (See chart on pp. 38–39)

Start now with the *physical gifts* you were given. Everyone is given a harvest of attributes that evolve over a lifetime. Whether it's a great head of hair, an awesome eye color, an expressive smile, pretty fingers, a stately nose, a curvaceous body, pretty feet, a cute nose, exotic features, full lips, smooth skin, pretty hair color, curly eyelashes, porcelain skin, chocolate skin, caramel skin, olive skin, attractive belly button, shiny hair, strong cheekbones, long forehead, interesting cowlicks, and on and on and on.

List your *physical attributes* on a separate piece of paper or the chart on the next page. If you have trouble with this, think about what others have complimented you on. Start with a minimum of ten.

Then we'll talk about *inner qualities*. What gifts were you given in that department? Patience, fortitude, insight, creativity, sensitivity, compassion, humor, strength, faith, trust, playfulness, honesty and understanding, clarity, openness, tenderness, efficiency, wisdom, flexibility?

If it helps to get started, you might use the words "I am" and then fill in the blank. It might look like this: I am beautiful, sexy, vulnerable. I am happy, successful, creative. I am precious, studious, disciplined. I am sensual, warm, compassionate. List a minimum of positive inner qualities.

Next, list your *unique gifts and talents.* Do you create beauty in every crevice of your home, nurture family members, bring out the courage in others, synthesize and clarify ideas, heal others from pain, create visions, execute details efficiently? Include ones you were born with and those you have honed. If you're a little fuzzy on the subject, consider what others have pointed out to you about yourself. Close your eyes and remember what they have said about you. Start again with a minimum of ten.

What are the *blessings in your life?* This is a gratitude list. What are those things that you are especially grateful for in your life, things that make your life particularly sweet and precious? Start you list. As you think of more things as the days and weeks go, add them.

What *resources* are available to you in your life? Do you have an education? Do you have supportive friends, a networking group, connections, guardian angels, s trust
fund, wise grandparents, friends in high places? Try to list at least ten.

Tell the truth. Especially now. With a little effort you will soon have long flowing lists of your personal assets. No stubby lists allowed! This may be the most important step you'll take to dressing yourself with joy, so don't think for a second about skipping over this part. You need the workout! I want to see your Focus on What Works muscle toned and responsive.

THE REASONS I WANT YOU TO FOCUS ON WHAT WORKS ARE:

1. **It's healthier.**

2. **It'll make you happier.**

3. **You'll know how to dress yourself.**

ATTRIBUTES	PHYSICAL GIFTS	INNER QUALITIES
wisdom		
awesome eyes		
creativity		
shiny hair		
humor		
cute nose		
openness		
olive skin		
fortitude		*flexible*
curly eyelashes		
faith		
strong cheek bones		
understanding		
expressive smile		
Patience		
pretty feet		
insight		
curvaceous body		
sensitivity		
long forehead		
compassion		
attractive belly button	*awesome eyes*	
strength		
exotic features		
trust		
porcelain skin		
playfulness		
chocolate skin		
honesty		
caramel skin		
clarity		
long neck		
tenderness		

GIFTS/TALENTS	BLESSINGS	RESOURCES
		networking group
artistic		
	my family	

GRAND TOTAL:

A wonderful YOU!

TRY THIS:

In your three-ring binder make a tab for Personal Assets (or Assets for short) or choose another word that fits better for you. In the Personal Assets section place copies of the lists you made in this exercise. If you prefer working on the computer, make your lists there, but print out some copies for your binder.

These lists are never finished. Keep adding to them. It's funny how quickly we forget the good stuff. I want the good stuff in front of you or near you at all times. Where's the good stuff? In your binder!

It wouldn't hurt to have copies in other places. You could have them on your nightstand, in your appointment book, in the drawer next to the refrigerator — somewhere nearby for when you take a quick five-minute pick-me-up break.

BUDDY EXERCISE:

Ask your buddy to write her own list of qualities she sees in you. Notice how fast and easy it comes to her. Are there things on your lists that are the same? Are there things you overlooked? Have your buddy listen for any clever ways you might have distorted a good thing into a bad thing, like "My neck isn't so bad given I'm such a chunky person."

Note to Buddies: If you smell negativity in the way your buddy has written her list, challenge her to re-focus on the positive. Remove anything that sounds negative, mean, or cruel.

Fashion Strategy #3: Stop Comparing

One day, when Roger, the computer repairman, was at my office, he told me that some of my files were corrupted. As women, the files in our heads get corrupted too. We're going to face one of our greatest vices: comparing. Some things are good to compare. Like mayonnaise brands. But comparing yourself to someone else as a way to feel superior or inferior is just no good. *Are you squirming yet?* This is one of women's ugliest secrets. It's automatic, rampant, incessant. And fixating. "If I was as thin as Carol, then I'd be okay. Well, I'm not as thin, but I am prettier." Or younger or richer or taller or brighter or more worldly or more talented or — you fill in the blank. Comparing is the evil twin to focusing on what doesn't work.

Women often place the foundation of their self-worth on a bed of sand that washes away when a beautiful woman walks through the door. Or they gather in small groups where they love to hate how attractive, accomplished, or athletic another woman is. It's a way women connect with other women. As a gender, if we're not picking on ourselves, we pick each other apart.

I've talked to many men about this. I've looked for evidence that this is something "humans" do, but I haven't found any. Men don't do this the way women do.

'Fess up. It may take you a while to notice you're doing it because you may be doing it unconsciously all the time. You may be comparing yourself every single time you meet someone. Before you open your mouth to say hello, you may look at a woman and think, "She has a beautiful smile and my teeth are crooked."

Oh, we laugh about this when we talk to our friends. "I went to yoga class and I met this woman," we say. "She's gorgeous. I hate her. And we're having lunch next Tuesday." Just how necessary is that "hating her" step? Why do we disapprove of someone because of their positive traits? What does that say about our relationship to our positive traits?

Think about it. It's not that funny. It breaks women down. Chipping away at each other diminishes our strength. If you make comparisons in your mind, or express them to others, you dishonor those women. This incessant comparison also dishonors yourself. It's as if we believe there is a scarcity of beauty in the world. There's plenty to go around. In fact, the more you notice beauty, the more beauty there is. Appreciating and accepting beauty in others doesn't deny it for you, it validates it for everyone.

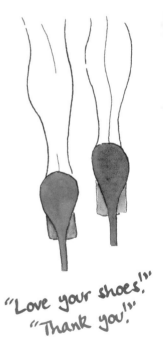

"Love your shoes!"
"Thank you!"

A compliment is the antidote to comparisons. Where comparisons diminish, compliments enhance. Be generous with each other instead of being stingy. Appreciate a woman's great hair or bubbly personality. And express that appreciation with a compliment: "You have the prettiest smile." Turn comparing into complimenting and see how beautiful YOU become!

Turn the art of complimenting into a habit. Jeanne, you do it in Tallahassee, Florida. Angela, you do it in Helena, Montana. Susan, you do it in Albany, New York. Margareta, you do it in Stockholm. Keiko, you do it in Hong Kong, and Brigitte, you do it in Paris. Then maybe we can turn this thing around.

Finally, recognize comparison for what it is. It's poison. You know how some people are allergic to shellfish? They break out in hives if they eat it. I want you to imagine breaking out in hives every time you're tempted to compare. Instead, practice compliments. Be generous with your appreciation. Compliment every single woman you talk to today. And then get up tomorrow and do it again.

A word about models: *Models are professional clothes hangers.* They make clothes look inviting. That's their job. Recently I saw a fashion spread in a magazine where attractive, thin women who had nothing to do with modeling, were modeling clothes. They were beautiful, but they weren't models and it showed. There are only about eight people in the world who look like models and get paid to do it. Well, maybe more than eight. But you are not one of them. You do something else. To expect your clothes to look like that on you is unrealistic. Do not compare yourself to models, think you are supposed to look like them, or believe that they are somehow the standard for women. They aren't. They are paid hangers. Leave them alone, let them do their jobs. Mind your own business.

It's revitalizing and rejuventating to remind yourself of your assets.

TRY THIS:
I bet you can think of three people who you thought about paying a compliment but for some reason you held back. Who in the last six months has really delighted you with their style or the way they've put colors together, or they way they accessorized an outfit? If you didn't compliment them at the time, it's not too late. Open up your heart, reach for a pen and make a list of those people who deserve a compliment from you. Formulate your thoughts. What did they do that got your attention? How did it make you feel? How did it impact your day or your mood or your thoughts? Now pick up the phone and call them and tell them what you've just been thinking about. Or send them a note. After you've complimented three people, check in with yourself and see how you feel. It feels good, doesn't it! Everyone benefits from compliments — the givers and the receivers.

Fashion Strategy # 4: Do the Love Thing

I want to know you're enjoying a life that holds beauty, ease, and pleasure. To do that, you have to make choices. From this moment on, feel compelled to choose only the things you love. When you are on aisle nine in the grocery store selecting tissues, pick the box design and tissue color that you LOVE. Not the one on sale, unless you happen to adore that one. Choose the one you LOVE. When you buy a new wallet, buy the one you love the feel of, the color of, the size of. Love the number of zippers, compartments, and slots it has. If you don't fall in love with that wallet, then leave the store empty-handed. Am I suggesting you wait? Yes. WAIT until you find a wallet that you LOVE. It's worth it. You're worth it. It's like a relationship. Every time you hold it you'll be glad you waited for the one you love.

When you are buying underwear, a running bra, a nightgown, a skirt, winter boots, a bathing suit, a wedding dress or an umbrella, buy the one you LOVE. Say NO to anything that isn't a YES. And don't ever say yes again when you mean no.

Maybe you are good at this in part of your life. You pick out the right silverware, bathroom mats, or frames for your family photos — ones you are happy with right from the start. But when it comes to clothes, you settle for what's on sale or what'll do. You think it doesn't matter. **It matters.** Wearing only clothes you love will certainly raise your life expectancy. Don't walk around in a "just-okay" wardrobe. It's lifeless, not fun, not exciting, not soothing, not even pleasant. Shape up your wardrobe with the "love" attitude.

LOVE MEANS:
NO lukewarm.
NO just okay.
NO it'll do.
There is only:
YES I love it!
YES I'm crazy about it!
YES it's perfect!

MAKE A LOVE LIST:

Write down everything that you're just crazy over. It doesn't have to be about clothes either. List anything that comes to your mind. You could love the look of something, the feel of something, the taste of something. Be specific. Slip into a love reverie and write down everything. You might have a list of fifty things (or more) so start here but proceed to your computer or another piece of paper if you need more space. Put the list in your binder when you have finished. Keep adding to it. See how big your heart can get.

Your list might include pink hydrangeas, cherry popsicles, watermelon in the summertime, the sound of crunching leaves in the fall, a calm lake, juniper trees, polka-dotted underwear, the color of cosmopolitans, the inside of Grace Cathedral. Start your list now.

I JUST LOVE IT:

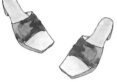

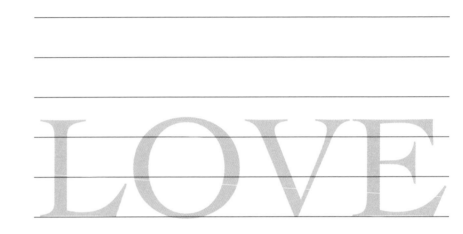

_____

_____

_____

_____

_____

_____

_____

BUDDY EXERCISE:

Make a research date with your buddy. Go to a gift store, jewelry store, or furniture store. Leave your cash and credit cards at home. This isn't about shopping to buy. Look for something you are wildly crazy about. Then pick out something you don't like at all and then something you're just lukewarm about. Point these three things out to your buddy and elaborate about what you love, what you hate, and what you're indifferent about. Trade off with your buddy and let her show you her picks. If you have time, do another round of this. You'll learn a lot about each other's tastes in this exercise, which will help you in the chapters ahead. The point is to appreciate each other's choices, not to agree on them. You and your buddy are different people and you'll have different picks.

Look around your bedroom. Are you surrounded by things you love? Ideally, if you share your bedroom with a mate, your mate is one of the things you love. Beyond that, are the pictures on the wall ones that you love? Do you love the color of your bedroom, the bedding, the rugs on the floor, the plants, the pulls on the dresser drawers? Tell the truth! If there are things there that you aren't crazy about get rid of them. Clear your visual space of anything that doesn't please you. If you're left with a mattress and a beautiful bedspread, be delighted. See what grows from being in love with it. Before you know it, the space begins to magically fill in with . . . you guessed it . . . only things that you love.

Fashion Strategy #5: Dress for the Body You Are Currently In

You know the body you're in right now? The one that's attached to the hands that are holding this book? That's the body I want you to dress. The one that's inhaling and exhaling as you skim these pages. Not the one you'd like to change or improve upon. Not the body you were in five years ago, or the one you fantasize about being in next year. It's time to adorn your precious body. This one.

I don't know a single woman who hasn't said, "When I lose weight, I'll go shopping, but not until then." Or they'll say something as silly as, "I won't buy anything if it's not a size 8." Good grief. Those are just numbers on tags! Your body wants to be happy in clothes now and it can be, right now, exactly as it is today.

One day I worked with Barbara. Her upper body wanted to live in ease in a size 14W or an OX. That's a different department to shop in than those she had shopped in before. She had great jackets in her closet that I was excited to work with, but the tops to go under them (the inside pieces) were all too skimpy. She needed different ones. She hesitated to go shopping. Instead, she thought she should change her body to fit into the old things in her closet.

You know the body you are in right now? The one that is holding this book? That's the one I want you to dress.

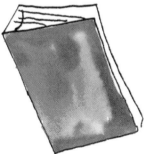

Her body had already changed. Her health had changed, and some medications she was taking were affecting her body size. To dress for the body she was currently in, she needed to visit another department. She didn't realize her struggle around clothes could magically disappear if she just strolled over to a women's department that held an extensive selection of items in her current size.

When I took her there, she was amazed. I knew she could look fabulous. She had been doubtful, but when she looked in the mirror, she exclaimed, "You mean I don't have to struggle anymore?"

Who wouldn't hate shopping if they constantly went to departments that didn't accommodate the body they were currently in? If where you shop makes you unhappy, shop somewhere else! Tell the truth. *Get current with your current body.*

This may sound elementary, but for many women it's a stumbling block. Here's the thing: a woman dressed in clothes that fit her gracefully radiates ease and confidence, while ill-fitting clothes make her look uncomfortable in her skin and her life. Choose ease and confidence, won't you? Let clothes support your being.

When babies outgrow their bassinets, we put them in a crib. We need to treat ourselves the same and handle our ongoing changes with good sense. Let go of your past lives as a teenager or a twenty-year-old or a thirty-year-old. Dress beautifully for the body you are currently in.

TRY THIS:
Go shopping for clothes that are two sizes bigger than you usually wear. Yes, you read that right. If you wear a size 10, try on a size 14. If you're wearing a 1X, try on a 3X. I want you to get rid of any historical obsession you might have with size or wearing a certain size.

Fashion Strategy #6: Think "Fit" First

This rule is a cozy next-door neighbor to Dress for the Body You Are Currently In. Because women focus so intensely on size, they lose all perspective on the lusciousness of good fit — good fit as a right, a requirement, a delight, something to expect, something to count on, long for, lust for, enjoy immeasurably, demand. I want to heighten your awareness of good fit so you insist on it every time you get dressed.

The way you know you're experiencing good fit is that you won't notice fit at all. No sleeves drag across your Caesar salad because they're hemmed to the right spot. You won't stand on the hem of your pants in your backless shoes because the pants will be hemmed properly. When you sit down, no prairie-dog mound of fabric will crowd your lap because your rise is a perfect length. *Bad fit gets your attention every time.* A bra with too-big cups too makes your sweaters look rumpled across your bra-line. A bra too narrow keeps you tugging on the underwire. Pants that ride up in the back keep you pulling the back seam out of your crack.

The beauty of good fit is that you never think about it because it works! I have a hard time getting sunglasses wide enough for my face and when I do, oh, it feels so good! Getting the seat of my bicycle adjusted to fit my legs just right is heavenly. Slipping into a pair of arms for a hug where everything lines up perfectly is so fine. Getting into someone's car whose passenger seat fits your back, bottom, and legs is yummy. Don't you want that for yourself in clothes? I do!

Women endure bad fit like they endure a bad job or a bad relationship. If you aren't enjoying good fit, you have to tell the truth. Would alterations make a difference? If not, let go and move on. Go out and buy a pair of black pants that fit! Or look for that new job, or for goodness sake, get a new boyfriend.

Sometimes good fit comes from knowing you can expect it. I love this quote by Edgar Watson Howe:

> *"A man has his clothes made to fit him;*
> *a woman makes herself fit her clothes."*

Men expect good fit and get it. They don't buy a suit and leave the store without having a tailor personalize the fit for them. Women aren't as well-trained, especially because they get so hung up on the size thing. Forget size! Go for fit. FIT FIRST.

Your body is unique — long in places, short in others, thinner in some, thicker in others. **Pay attention to its geometry.** For some, tops from the petite department will fit best, while pants from the regular women's department will accommodate a longer rise. If you're short-waisted, you may opt to take waistbands off your skirt

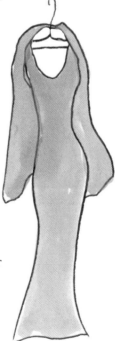

and pants. Or if you like having your pants sit high on your waist, you may add belt loops so that pants stay up. Or you may choose a little shoulder pad because your shoulders are narrow and it balances your hips.

Ladies, learn a thing or two from men. Expect to make alterations, expect to take things in, up, off, out in order to get good fit. If something doesn't fit you, it's not your body's fault, it's the garment's fault. Try on twenty pairs of jeans, sixteen sweaters, or fifty-five bras until you get the fit that you love. Remember, bad fit gets your attention like a mosquito in a darkened bedroom at midnight. Good fit gets no attention at all.

BUDDY EXERCISE:

Almost everyone has an area of her body that is really easy to fit, plus one that is hard to fit (or so they say). Make a "hard-to-fit" area the focus of a shopping expedition. Get some professional opinions on fit. Try to shop at a store that has in-store alterations staff. Try on lots of whatever is hard to fit on you — jeans, blouses, bathing suits (yes!), skirts. Ask the salesperson for help in fitting the area you're working on. A good salesperson really understands that one pant runs long, another short. Or a waistband is wider or narrower on different brands. Shop with success in mind. When you're really close to finding a good fit, call in an alterations person and see if they can suggest adjustments for an even better fit. Come home with a success fit story and share it with your buddy. You will learn a lot about fit just by trying lots of things on, asking questions, and getting a tailor's support. Everyone can enjoy great fit!

Fashion Strategy #7: You're Worth Full Price

May I say right now that you're worth full price? Just take that in, sit quietly, close your eyes, and listen to this — you're worth full price. I love springing this idea on women, especially those addicted to sales and bargain prices. Sometimes bargain-hunting pays, but it carries a subtle and often unconscious message that's saying "I'm not worth full price." This can slide awfully fast to "I'm not valuable." So, let's get a few things straight: When you learn how to identify and satisfy your clothing needs with the right choices, it becomes much less important what it costs. I want you to **wear what you love and love what you wear.** When you do that, you get your money's worth.

Way too often I find an item in a client's closet that still has the "great deal" price tag attached and has never been worn. The price tag was satisfying in some way, but the garment didn't move the satisfaction meter in the buyer's heart. Sometimes we buy five cheap blouses trying to find the satisfaction that a single more expensive blouse would provide — one we'd always wear. While the other five hang quietly in the closet, we remain dissatisfied and long for the one we left behind.

Go for what you love and pay the price because you're worth it. And wear for wear, it's worth it! You didn't get any value out of the five blouses you bought (and didn't wear) that added up to one hundred dollars. If you'd bought the hundred dollar blouse that you loved and wore it one hundred times, the cost per wear was one dollar. Now that's a bargain.

If you get that value from your bargains, that's great. But if you aren't, then blast your shopping style with this strategy and see if your satisfaction with your clothes soars.

SO, LET'S GET A FEW THINGS STRAIGHT:

1. You're not cheap.

2. You are as precious as pure gold.

3. You are worth spending money on.

4. Your needs are worth being met.

TRY THIS:
Take a shopping field trip. Go to a store that sells clothes that are priced beyond what you've ever spent before. Study the clothes, inside and out. What do you love about the fabric, cut, or color? Look at the price. Try something on. See how it feels to be inside full price clothes that are also pricier than you are used to wearing. I'm not suggesting you buy anything. I'm just asking you to bypass the "sale/discount" mental state and ponder how it feels to be worth full price.

Fashion Strategy # 8: Don't Save Good Clothes for "Good" — Good Is Right Now

NANCY had this top she just loved, a lime-green satin blouse in a lively print featuring martini glasses tipped at different angles. After she bought it, it hung in her closet for months. Because the fabric was shiny, she thought it should be for special occasions and kept waiting for a special time to wear it. One day she thought: I love this blouse. I

What are you
waiting for?
Don't save
your clothes,
WEAR THEM!

love how I feel when I wear it. *I'm just going to wear it NOW!* And she did — to work, the grocery store, the movies. She was so happy! Wearing it reminded her that "special" is right now.

If you buy clothes and then wait six to twelve months to rip off the tags and start wearing them, you're not alone. It's curious. Some clients say new clothes have to mingle and mellow in their closets before they are ready to be worn. Or they'll say, "The new clothes are so good, I can't wear them right away." Don't save good clothes for good — "good" is right now. There, I said it again and I hope it will hasten your process from buying to wearing.

Clothes are expensive. They are an investment. **Get your money's worth right away.** Rip off the tags, slip into your new duds, and prance yourself out the door into the sunshine of your day.

IF YOU DON'T, YOU RUN THE RISK OF:

Forgetting that they are there

Waiting so long that they go out of style

Postponing tons of joy that you could
be experiencing inside of those clothes

Asking yourself nine months later,
"Why did I wait so long?"

TRY THIS:

Walk into your closet. Open up your jewelry box. Pull out your lingerie drawer. Select five things you have been saving "for good" — a necklace your mom gave you, a beaded sweater, a velvet coat, a lacy nightgown. Plan to wear those things next week. If you think you don't have any place to wear a given item, make something up! Plan a dinner party. Invite someone on a date. Create an evening out with your buddy so she can come in one of her "good" outfits. See how much fun you can have.

One Giant Leap

Remember when I said that practicing just one fashion strategy would change your life? I bet you're feeling it right now. Have you had an ah-ha or two or three or twenty? If you get your mind to focus on what works, acknowledge the blessings in your life, and counter your comparisons with compliments, you're on your way to being a much happier, freer woman who can truly enjoy getting dressed and being satisfied with her clothes every day. If you keep around you only what you love and joyfully, without judgment, dress your body as it is right now, putting "fit first" every time, your shopping abilities take a giant leap forward. In no time, you'll have a closet full of best friends. Everything in there will work. Can you feel how effortless this is becoming and you haven't even stepped into your closet yet!

And now that you know you're worth full price, you've increased the bank account of your self-worth exponentially. Realizing that "good" is right now means you'll be getting so much more value from your wardrobe. I'm so happy for you! Your fashion strategies are the wind at your back, making everything that follows much easier to accomplish.

In the next chapter you're going to go deeper into your past, examining your history with shopping for and wearing clothes. By *re*viewing the past, you can let go of habits that don't serve you well and gain ones that will serve you better. You'll listen, let go, and

create a new plan!

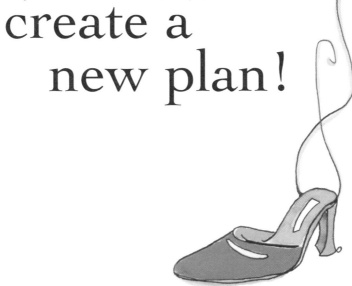

Going Deeper

IF YOU DON'T HAVE ISSUES involving clothes, you're one lucky, unusual gal. Most of us have survived in spite of misguided outfits salespeople talked us into, mean school kids who picked on anyone who looked "different," teasing brothers who made fun of our looks, or the prom dress nightmare that left us mortified. If you didn't get bad clothing advice growing up, you probably got no clothing advice at all. I don't think anyone leaves childhood or adolescence without clothing issues that linger and get in the way of having a fret-free wardrobe.

The Issues

There are plenty of reasons to be hung up about clothes, body image and how we felt about these things growing up. Here are some issues women have shared with me.

DEBORAH never had new clothes of her own, but wore hand-me-downs from a cousin who was a foot taller and wider than she was. VALERIE'S mother left the family when Valerie was young, and her clothing advice came from her dad, who didn't have a clue. JOAN, at sixteen, changed to a new school where students didn't wear uniforms. When Joan's mom took her shopping for school clothes, she bought her outfits appropriate to a forty-year-old, not a teenaged daughter. LINDA grew up being teased unmercifully for being chubby. MOLLY grew up being teased unmercifully for being skinny. JENNY was molested as a child and feared clothes for the attention they could bring to her body. SUSAN got the message loud and clear that her father wished she'd been a boy. TRACY'S parents were missionaries in an impoverished country, and her love of fashion was a passion she needed to keep secret. ALICE felt misplaced because she wanted to dress like a New York sophisticate while growing up in rural Iowa. CAROLYN was raised with all brothers, and her mother dressed her just like them.

ABBY'S parents, profoundly affected by the Depression, instilled the value in her that you never throw anything away.

Your clothing issues from the past are affecting your current wardrobe experience. By looking back, we'll see how those issues are influencing you today. To create a new future, it's important to clear out the past.

Even though the circumstances of your life have changed, often those issues from "way back when" still run your life today. Once you separate yourself from what was "then," you can freely embrace "now."

Tell someone what happened when you were a girl. Really tell someone all about it. Call up your buddy or grab your notebook, or get a circle of friends together and share your experiences. Sharing them will help you breathe a big sigh of relief. It may even bring a tear or two. It helps to see the source of your patterns. When you get some distance from them, you come closer to having what you want in your life now. You'll be able to make new choices, something you may not have had the chance to do when growing up.

I have a list of questions to get you started. Feel free to improvise. Let your stories flow like water from a faucet. Expand your capacity for compassion. Feel compassion not only toward others, but also experience compassion for yourself — that's what I'm looking for here.

Grab a chunk of time and explore these questions either by talking with someone else or by writing about them in your journal.

SHARE YOUR EXPERIENCES: When you get distance from them, you come closer to having what you want in your life now.

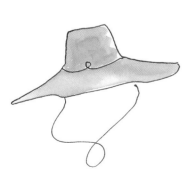
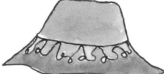
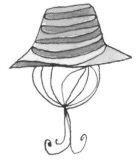

QUESTIONS:

1. Who took you shopping? Was the person a good shopper?

2. What did you learn about shopping from that person?

3. Where did your clothes come from? Did you baby-sit to earn money to buy your own clothes?

4. What was shopping like?

5. Did you or your mother sew your clothes? Was that successful?

6. Did you wear hand-me-downs? How did that work out for you?

7. Did you have what you needed — clothes for all kinds of activities and all kinds of weather? Did you have proper underwear and did you pick it out?

8. Did you shop sales? Did you shop only during sale times?

9. Did you like clothes?

10. Did you talk about clothes with your girlfriends? Go shopping together? Call each other up and talk about what you were wearing to school the next day?

11. Did you trade clothes with your friends?

12. Did anyone ever make fun of what you wore?

13. Did you have vivid dreams about clothes?

14. Did religion play a part in how you dressed?

15. If you had more than one mom (or other relatives who were responsible for shopping for you), did their styles and attitudes about clothes differ, and how did that affect you?

16. Did you have big swings in having clothes and not having them? Periods of time when your family had money for such things and times when they didn't?

17. Were you in the "in" crowd in high school?

18. Were you known for your style?

19. Were you known for your lack of style, or your style rebellion?

20. Were you part of a group in high school who had a certain "look"?

21. Were you ever punished for not keeping your room neat where the punishment involved your clothes being taken or given away? Or by having all your clothes pulled out of drawers and thrown on the floor?

22. Did your mother buy you clothes you didn't need or refused to wear?

23. Did your mother buy you things she liked and you didn't? Did you get your say in your clothing choices?

24. Did you and your family members dress in matching outfits?

25. Did you borrow clothes from your sisters?

26. Did your sister borrow clothes from you? How did that turn out?

27. Did your mother let you wear her jewelry?

When you discuss your early years of getting dressed with your buddy, or another friend, here are some things I want you and your friend to do:

Listen to each other's stories with no desire to fix anything. Everyone has a story to tell. Graciously receive each other's story.

Don't compare stories in a competitive way.

TRY THIS:

1. BORROW FROM OTHERS

Did you hear things in other's stories that you'd like to adopt in your life? Feel at liberty to ask someone for more details if there is a seed in her story you'd like to harvest for yourself. Someone's great experience shopping with her father could inspire a new way for you to think about shopping. Feel free to borrow. We are throwing a bunch of ideas out into the middle of the floor. Treat them like clothes and take what works for you. Look for the things you love and want to have in your life now.

2. LET YOUR STORY BE TOLD

If you have a traumatic childhood clothing story, share it with your buddy. Once we've told our stories and feel like we've really been heard, it's easier to move on. Your buddy is there to really listen. She can be your witness as you clarify what you no longer want to be running your life.

The Moth Story

You're a big girl now. All grown up. You get to keep what works and throw out the rest. We can't erase our past, but we can change our minds about it and replace what needs replacing.

I left North Dakota and moved to California when I was eighteen. On one of my visits home, I walked into my bedroom with my mom right ahead of me. She let out a scream when she saw a moth in the window. I was afraid of moths too. If there was one in my room, growing up on the farm, I couldn't sleep. Seeing my mother react like this made me realize that my fear of moths started with her. I thought

We can't erase our past, but we can change our minds about it and replace what needs replacing.

about it for a minute. Was I really afraid of those small critters? No. I learned this fear. **I realized right then I had a choice in the matter.** Now I love moths. They fascinate me.

Do you have a "moth" story in your life? Are there things you picked up from others that you have a choice about? What are you doing in your life now that really doesn't fit for you? What inherited beliefs no longer serve you?

You can have a totally different experience than you had as a kid. Moms have lots of skills, but knowing about clothes isn't always one of them. I'm here to be the shopping mom you wish you had. This workbook is here to give you a new experience.

Start creating that new experience by coming up with some statements that will be your guidelines. What loving statements can you make that when you read them will guide you toward a new and improved relationship to clothes? Include everything you want for yourself at this time. Borrow from other people's success if you heard some success stories. Make affirming statements that you can really live with comfortably for the next few months. And then revise them as you get more experience. Call this your vision.

EXAMPLE:

I please myself in clothing. Everything I wear makes me feel great. I take the time I need to shop. I listen to other's opinions, but I have the final say. I love to go shopping.

After you've written your vision, talk it over with your buddy. She may have some points on her list you may want to add to yours.

MY VISION/MY WAY/MY SAY:

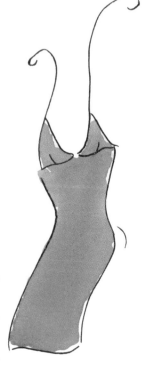

_____

_____

_____

To Cling is to Suffer

Now that we've identified some patterns you inherited from your past, let's move on to some things you may have created all on your own. There's something women do that creates an endless number of aches and pains. What is it? Clinging. You know how clinging feels, right? It's that gnawing feeling in your gut. A boyfriend has broken up with you, moved to New England, and you keep clinging to the relationship. The more you cling, the more it keeps you from being present and getting on with your life.

A big source of pain for some people is to ache over something they don't have but see in others — like good muscle tone, a trim waistline, great hair, a certain bra or dress size — or over what they once had and then lost. In either case, we cling to what was or what we wish could be. It's all clinging. The result is suffering. When we indulge that ache, we lose out on enjoying what we do have.

Focusing on what you cling to can come across your radar screen once a day, twelve times a day, or maybe even obsessively. What do you cling to?

HERE ARE A FEW PLACES WHERE WOMEN CLING:

Being a size 8

Growing up with natural blond hair that isn't natural anymore

Being ten pounds lighter

Not having youthful flawless skin

Perky pre-children breasts

Attention for a once shapely figure

Okay. Make your own list. Do you spend time fretting over things you lost or things you wish you had but don't? Tell the truth. Don't leave anything out. Write until there's nothing left to write.

> You know how clinging feels, right? It's that gnawing feeling in your gut . . . the more you cling, the more it keeps you from being present and getting on with your life.

I'M CLINGING TO:

_____

_____

_____

Nothing stays the same. That we can count on. Your most prized possessions could disappear — a waistline, a thick head of hair, eyebrows, flawless skin, shapely legs — but the whole of you remains.

How do we deal with these losses? We mourn them. We cry, get angry, or bargain — if we can just get that waist back, we'll never eat chocolate again. After all that fails (and it will) then it's time to accept what is and be grateful for what we have.

Appreciate What You Have

Using the Tell-the-Truth-Let Go-Create mantra, it's time to create appreciation for what you have. While you can do this exercise on your own, I recommend doing it with your buddy or a trusted friend. Look at your facial features, your coloring, your body and the general first impressions you make. For each of these areas, write down three things you like. Ask your buddy to do the same assignment with you in mind. Review both lists. These are the areas that you can play up and accentuate when getting dressed. Let's begin. What facial features do you want to bring into focus?

What are your best features? What kinds of clothes would highlight those features?

BEST FEATURES:

_____

_____

_____

Wearing what colors would bring out your natural radiance? Look at your hair, skin and eyes.

BEST COLORS:

_____

_____

_____

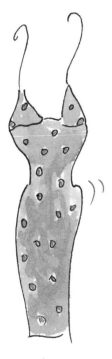

What part of your body would be great to emphasize? Hands, shoulders, waist, bust, hips, bottom, legs, etc.

BODY HIGHLIGHTS:

_____

_____

_____

What kinds of clothes would highlight those body parts? For example, a boat neck sweater shows off a long, straight shoulder line; short skirts show off great legs; a low-cut V-necked sweater shows off a pretty bust line.

CLOTHING HIGHLIGHTS:

_____

_____

_____

What are some general first impressions you make to others? For example: dramatic, dynamic, innocent, sweet, sophisticated, witty.

FIRST IMPRESSIONS:

_____

_____

_____

It's much more efficient to spend your time, energy, and money on highlighting what you already have here and now. You already have great features, unique coloring, and personality traits that are all your own. Pay attention to what you have and find ways to bring it to your own (and others') attention by wearing colors that are good on you, by wearing clothes that highlight your best features, by putting an exclamation point on one of your personality traits — like wearing bright playful prints to accentuate your witty side. Celebrate yourself. Don't fret over what you don't have. Celebrate what you do have!

Name That Rut

You realize newfound freedom when you shift attention away from perceived flaws and focus on your assets. So we're ready to look at another place where we get stuck: our ruts. Everyone's got them. It's like mosquitoes in Minnesota in July — you can't avoid them. Your ruts have names: all black, all the time; one thousand pairs of khakis with no distinctions; always in jeans; living in sweats; 1980s hair; plucked-to-nothing eyebrows.

HERE'S WHAT'S TRUE ABOUT RUTS:

There's not one drop of creativity in a rut. Any creativity that was initially there is now dried up, caked and flaky.

RUTS
You know you've got 'em. Be brave and admit them now. What are your ruts?

There's no thought in a rut. That's what makes it a rut. It's a habit. Like putting on the same ratty bathrobe at 5:17 P.M. when you get home from work.

There's no courage in a rut. Also no adventure, no excitement - it's lifeless.

NAME YOUR RUTS:

_____

_____

_____

_____

Pink? Lace? Sheer? See which ones make you feel happy, sexy, satisfied.

There are antidotes to ruts. The first step to get out of your ruts is to catch yourself heading toward them. When you're in the lingerie department and go for the same pair of undies you've worn for thirty years, ask yourself if those undies are really satisfying. If when you think about it, your heart hangs down around your belly button and your shoulders cave in, the answer is no. If your heart rests high in your chest and you feel expansive when you hold those panties in your hand, then the answer is yes. *Listen to your heart.* Tell the truth. Let go of your rut. *Create a new response* — one that thrills you. Look through the rows of panties and see what calls to you now. Pink? Lace? Jockeys? Sheer ones? Thongs? Gather lots of undies. Go to a dressing room and try them on (over your own undies) and see which ones make you feel happy, sexy, satisfied.

If you have a tough time, pick up the phone and call your buddy. That's what she's there for. "Hey, Buddy, guess where I am?" you'll say. "Standing in front of the white cotton panties bin and feeling bad. These aren't me! Talk to me before I come home with a baker's dozen!"

Look at your ruts and brainstorm alternatives. Let your buddy give you input. List each rut and come up with some action to get you out of them. Ask your buddy to help you. If your rut is always wearing black, your action step is to focus on other colors.

RUT: ACTION:

_____   _____

_____   _____

_____   _____

_____   _____

_____   _____

_____   _____

Good Job! Congratulations! You're stronger now. When you separate yourself from the habits and beliefs that don't support you, you're free to discover yourself anew. And boy, I've got some great ways for you to do that! Say bye-bye to the past. Get ready to ride the Ferris wheel of fun as you **find the style that's right for you now.**

Get the Picture

NOW YOU KNOW where your personal land mines are and you have some tools for deploying them. You're ready to defend against those nagging aches and pains with clothes, rooted in the past. After your long look backward and into the present, it's time to shine a big spotlight in front of you so you can see what lies ahead: your wonderful new life in clothes without hang-ups or restrictions.

I've found the best way to do this is with images, imagination, and visualization. We're going to start out with some collage work because you don't do much thinking with collages. You just do them. They're fast and more fun than art class in first grade.

You have a diamond mine inside you and collages are a way to reach those gems. Cutting out images and words and arranging them on a piece of paper is worth twelve months of therapy and six months of career counseling. It's quick. It's illuminating. It's like waking up from a beautiful dream that gave you all the answers to a problem that almost kept you up all night.

Making collages can help you visualize how you'd like to look in clothes. They will clarify the parts of yourself you want to express now. You may be very surprised!

You've probably made a collage before. Maybe you've "collaged" the new year by making a treasure map of all the things you wanted to have happen in that year. One client did a treasure map every December and put it on a wall in her bathroom where she'd be reminded of the things she wanted in her life. There's nothing like waking up in a fog and feeling blue, hardly remembering your name, let alone your plan for life, then glancing over at a collage you made and BOOM! — you remember.

Oh yeah! THAT'S where I'm going!

If you've never made a collage, it's easy. All you need is a stack of magazines on architecture, gardening, fashion, health, travel, lifestyle, movies, whatever! They don't have to be current issues, at least not for the first exercise. You need scissors, a glue stick, and a poster or mat board to mount your images on. Carve out a chunk of time — either a full afternoon, evening, or a weekend slot. If you find yourself needing more time than you thought, give it to yourself.

You can also do this project with your buddy. Share magazines and plan to make a big mess. Put on your favorite music and work quietly side-by-side. Save your feedback until the end.

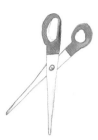

Collage Rules and Regs

To begin, quickly page through magazines or catalogs looking for images to rip out. Don't stop to read the articles. If you're tempted to check out an article, rip it out, and set it aside in a "reading" pile for later. Rip out images or words that appeal to you. Enjoy that ripping sound.

Let the unconscious part of you take the wheel. Don't think about what you're doing. Paging through magazines and ripping out images gets you far, far away from your head. I don't want to know what you think. I want to know what you feel. If, in any of these exercises, you pick things for someone else's approval or to fulfill an expectation, throw those out. But if other people's ideas — like your husband's, mom's, sister's, or best friend's — are crowding your head, then go ahead and pull them and put those in a separate pile. Get that out of the way so you can go on to satisfying yourself. Later you can show the "other people" pile to your buddy, if you'd like, and tell her the stories around them. It'll help you draw a good distinction between what's "you" and how other people view you.

After you've ripped through the magazines, trim the images to remove any unnecessary part of the picture. Then gather up all your images and spread them out on a wide surface like a dining room table, kitchen counter, coffee table, or the floor. Sort through the images. If you find images that don't resonate as strongly the second time through, toss them. Stick to the ones that really zing for you. Be picky. You can always go back for more images if you need to. Now that you understand the basics, let's begin.

**PULL OUT ANY-
THING THAT:**

- **You just love**
- **You want more of**
- **You admire in others**
- **Inspires you**
- **Appeals to you for no conscious reason at all**

From Pictures to Style

I've got three activities up my red-cardiganed sleeve. Decide which ones you want to do alone and which ones you want to do with your buddy.

I Just Want to Be Me

This collage exercise will help you discover what is hidden inside of you. That's the beauty of collage and manipulating images. When you take one image and lay another alongside it, it may produce a feeling that is more powerful for you than any feeling the pieces could have produced individually. It's that combustible energy that you are looking for. With this exercise you will begin to create your own language out of symbols that are meaningful to you.

STEP 1 Gather up your supplies — magazines, catalogs, scissors, paper, and a glue stick.

STEP 2 Close your eyes, sit comfortably in a chair with your feet on the ground and think about these questions: Who have I become? What wants to be expressed right now? What's inside of me that's just aching to come out? Where is my passion right now?

STEP 3 Hold these questions in your heart and go through a stack of magazines (they don't have to be current ones). Rip out images and phrases that give the answers. Trust yourself. I want to see paper flying everywhere. Don't labor over this. MOVE — don't think!

STEP 4 Trim your images. Start arranging the images on a mat board in a way that means something to you, or is pleasant or appealing, or that just compels you in some way. Don't work too hard at this. If you look at the images on the page and they don't stir you, you're not there yet. Keep moving them around until they sizzle with energy or strike a deep chord in you.

You may have started out making one collage, but then it seemed to want to splinter off into a few smaller ones. That's okay too. Let the collages have their way. Once the pieces are arranged to your liking, get a glue stick and stick them to the page.

STEP 5 Let the images speak to you. Now that you have collected and arranged the images on a page, look at them closely. I realize that what you are looking at may be hard to put in words, but try to verbalize

If you look at the images on the page and they don't stir you, you're not there yet. Keep moving . . .

what you see. This is where your buddy can be a big help. Talk about the images. Let your buddy ask you clarifying questions about it. See if you can identify qualities that the collage represents. Are you seeing parts of yourself that have been hidden from view? A strength? A determination? A softness? A vulnerability? What is the overall feeling that comes from your collage?

Meet Maggie. When Maggie, an efficient, professional, no-nonsense woman looked at her collage, she said it was like looking down a deep well. What she saw in the images was her womanliness, softness, and vulnerability. I asked her if she felt ready to express those qualities in her life. She answered enthusiastically, "Yes! Absolutely! At last!"

STEP 6 "Read" your images. If you can't find words for them yet, that's okay. Collages are like dreams. Images have a distinctive language. Sit with your collage. It will continue to reveal itself to you over time. Eventually the words will come, and when they do write them here.

Pictures will bring to the surface what you love faster than my asking you if you like pink or lavender, or leather or satin.

_____

_____

_____

_____

_____

_____

_____

Enjoy your images. Absorb them. Their message will be a tremendous guide when you're putting clothes together in your closet. Put your collages in your binder.

The Looks I Love Today

In this exercise, the images you select will help give you specific direction in putting your look together. Choose the colors you are mad about. Let an accessory have its way with you. Allow a combination of separates to suddenly make perfect sense.

STEP 1 Go through a stack of current fashion magazines and catalogs (like the last three months). Pull out pictures of anything that you LOVE. I don't care if the price tag on the item is $14,000. You aren't buying it, you're just loving it. So rip it out and put it in a pile.

STEP 2 Go through the pictures and be sure you resonate with them all. Sometimes people pull pictures because they are afraid they won't get enough of them. They pull things that are close but not really hitting the right spot. If you only have three pictures that you LOVE, I will be happy. Don't worry about quantity. Quality is key. Don't question what you have pulled.

Meet Beth. Beth pulled pictures with very strong clues about her femininity. There were lots of dresses, lots of baby blue colors, lots of lace. The day we were looking at the pictures together she was dressed in black slacks, black lace-up shoes, and a blue shirt (men's style) tucked in. She had no jewelry on whatsoever. The pictures we were looking at looked completely different from the woman sitting there with me in the coffee shop. When I asked Beth what she loved about the pictures, she gushed about the femininity. And then she quickly pointed out, "But that's not me." And I said, "But if you could bring these qualities into your life, would you be happy?" And she said, "Well, yes, but I guess I never thought about doing such a thing. You know, my father always wanted me to be a boy." I asked her, "Would you like to look more like the women in these pictures?" And she said, "Could I?" "Absolutely," I reassured her. After our shopping trip, Beth was the perfect picture of femininity in pastels, dresses, and lace and she was thrilled.

STEP 3 Talk about what you love in your pictures. One by one, look at them and be specific about what attracts you. See if any patterns arise. Put like things together in separate piles. If you find you've pulled lots of pictures of necklaces, group them. If you have lots of pictures of monochromatic outfits (outfits that are all in shades of one color) group them. If you see a pattern of lively colors in playful clothes, group those.

STEP 4 Pretend you are a fashion editor. You've been given all these pictures and told to look at them all and report on the trends you are seeing. Start recording your comments. Better yet, have your buddy listen as you talk and she can write what you say. Before long you'll see that you have some themes going here. You might hear yourself saying, "I love these long, clean lines in clothes." Or "I love these shiny buttons." Or "I love these luxury fabrics." Or "It's the sheer flowing stuff that sends me." Or "I love solids." "Give me simple design." "Lots of texture soothes me." "I'm crazy for bold geometric patterns." "I love really homey, comfortable looks, nothing high-fashion or stiff."

STEP 5 Report on the trends that you see. If you have picked two or more pictures of similar things (bold colors, lacey fabrics, unusual prints), then you have a trend started. That trend is part of your new look. List those looks.

LOOKS I LOVE:

_____

_____

_____

_____

_____

_____

Put it on paper so you can identify it later when you are in a store. Now you know more about what you love and you can ask for what you want.

What Would Bridget Wear?

Here's an exercise for discovering a latent part of yourself that is ready to come out of the closet and get dressed. But first a story. I remember the first day I met Persia's new cat, Shirley (Yes, Persia is my friend and Shirley is her cat.). I'd already heard a lot about the cat — how she walked with a wiggle because something was wrong with her spine. When I entered the living room, she sauntered diagonally across my path, her backside twisting to the left like a fish's tail in a bucket, only slower and a lot prettier. This pet was definitely feminine. Persia had had her for less than a week and wasn't sure if she wanted to keep her original name. This cat was no Shirley, I'm telling you. Persia was debating over naming her Sammie after a favorite aunt, or Zsa Zsa. Watching that cat swish across the room to reach the thick velvet bronze drapes at the other end was all we needed to do to convince us she was Zsa Zsa. It suited her personality and style. Zsa Zsa she is.

Meet Bridget

Let me introduce you to Bridget. Bridget's name is actually Barbara, which is a perfectly fine name, but a few months ago I persuaded Barbara to play with a pseudonym that would help tweak her clothing style. She was in a rut. She hadn't been excited by her clothes in months — no, years, she admitted. I asked her to think about the qualities she wanted to bring out in herself. She was having a hard time naming qualities so I proposed a name change. I said, "What if there was a name that matched the qualities you'd like to be bringing out right now?" I asked. She quickly answered, "Bridget." "Great," I said, "so let's think about what Bridget would wear. Got some ideas?"

"Well, yeah," Barbara said. "Bridget is spunky, sassy. She's real, not pretentious. *She doesn't worry so much about what's appropriate.* She's more interested in being true to herself. She's sexy but not slutty. She's playful and carefree but not careless. She speaks her mind and doesn't worry about being perfect."

I asked Barbara if her wardrobe at home matched Bridget's. "No way!" Barbara said. "I've got 'nice' trousers and 'okay' sweaters. Nothing spicy enough for Bridget. She'd look at my closet and yawn."

While Barbara was fading into the woodwork, Bridget didn't mind getting some attention. Barbara's "nice" trousers got replaced by some flattering Bridget pants (not baggy or drapey, but snugger, more body conscious) in prints and in textures. The lace-up oxfords were replaced by stretch red leather boots that hugged the ankle and calf and had a two-and-a-half-inch heel. She also bought slides that showed off pretty painted toes. Barbara hadn't thought about showing off her toes, but Bridget did.

Now Bridget might not be the aspect of herself that Barbara brings to a board meeting — she still has those nice trousers and cardigan sets for that — but Bridget may have a say in the underwear Barbara puts on that day. When Barbara is not sure what to wear, she'll ask herself, "What would Bridget wear?"

SO, who's inside you who wants to get dressed and come out and play?

WHO'S INSIDE YOU?

I don't know how you feel about your name, but what if you could choose a new one? Is there a name that is better suited to you now? What name fits for you?

With your alter ego's name in mind, go through magazines and pull out pictures of things that she'd wear. You may not adopt the whole look of your Bridget, but you may adopt parts of it. What do you see from the pictures you've pulled that you'd like to try?

TRY IT

BUDDY EXERCISE:
Take your alter egos shopping. Try on clothes that "Bridget" likes to wear. Have fun dressing each other's persona. Don't stop until your buddy exclaims, "There's Bridget!" Dressing your alter ego helps you get out of your own way. It helps you bypass your critical voice that says, "You can't do THAT!" Maybe YOU couldn't, but Bridget can. This can crystallize what's been vague and hard to define about your personal style.

Create "My Style Words"

I asked you to make collages without thinking, to just go for what you loved. Now pull out the other part of your brain — the analytical part. Review your work. Collect all the "style words" that have come up throughout these exercises and write them down in the My Style Words box. By style words, I mean those words that describe your essence and preferences. Expect to collect anywhere from four to ten words.

Do a little review. While you were looking at the images in the Looks I Love exercise, what were the common threads? Distill those words and add them to your style words. When you did the What Would Bridget Wear exercise, what additional words came up to describe parts of you you'd like to express now? Add those too. In this space, collect all the words that describe what you've discovered about your style.

MY STYLE WORDS:

_____

_____

_____

_____

_____

_____

_____

STYLE WORDS
Elegant
Sophisticated
Playful
Alluring
Original
Delicate
Soft
Strong
Confident
Dramatic
Whimsical
Ladylike
Beautiful

JUST FOR FUN:

Did you ever play restaurant when you were a kid? I did. My two older brothers and I made a restaurant in our backyard one summer. We designed a menu making sure we could serve the things on it before we invited our parents to dine. One of us was the cook, one was the waiter and one was the host. It was so much fun.

Maybe you played beauty parlor and gave shampoos, haircuts and new hairstyles to your pets, teddy bears or younger siblings.

You're a grownup now but I invite you to play magazine publisher in that same delightful way you role-played professions as a kid. Create a magazine that's all about you. Its title could be your name, or maybe you'd want to use your alter ego's name. Put everything in that magazine that is all about you — what you love to do, what you love to wear, where you love to travel. Put it in a binder or buy a big spiral journal to store the pages. Design the cover. Fill the inside with pictures of things you love and places you want to visit. Write editorial pieces too. Or you could write a feature article about your alter ego. Write a tribute to those who have supported you along your path. Write an article on all the things you love to do in your leisure time.

Make it look like a real magazine. If you're clever on the computer you can do a great layout and scan pictures. Otherwise, do as we did as kids and keep it simple. Get creative. Get messy. Have a ball. This is a real treasure piece to keep forever. If we meet each other, I would love to see your personal magazine!

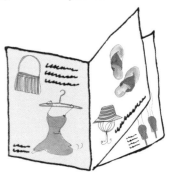

BUDDY EXERCISE:

This is a "My Favorite Things" exercise where you look for non-clothing clues to your fashion style. Each of you choose three objects from home that you absolutely love. Then get together for show and tell. As you describe what you love about each item, have your buddy write down what you say. See what words pop out. Capture the words that elicit strong visual images — words like whimsical, elegant, sleek, complex, simple, luxurious, refined, symmetrical, quiet, loud, bold, strong. Your buddy could be describing a teacup, a piece of art, a quilt, a vase, a bracelet, a mug. Listen carefully as she speaks from her heart about her love for each object. The words she uses often reveal helpful style words. They may also reveal looks she loves. Read back to her the words or looks you captured. They may be similar for each object. Ask her if she'd like those qualities in her clothes, or if those qualities were in her clothes now, would she be happy about it? Chances are she would love to reflect those qualities. Good harvesting! Ask her to add those to her style words list.

From Words to Style

We've been focusing on how clothes express the uniqueness of you — right now. You created words to describe your style. I'll be referring to those words as your style recipe.

SOME SAMPLE STYLE RECIPES FROM MY CLIENTS:

Sally: simple, clean, quiet, comfortable, soothing

Carol: mysterious, quirky, delightful, relaxed, luxurious

Margaret: girlie, sweet, natural, vibrant

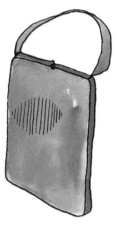

I LOVE IT.

Once you have your style recipe, you will take it into the closet or dressing room and use it as your guide when selecting clothes and accessories. Every look you build will incorporate some of your style words.

Take SALLY. When Sally puts together an outfit, she uses her style recipe. Let's build an outfit for her using "clean" and "quiet," two of her style words. What we would NOT choose would be a bright floral-print cropped T-shirt with pink corduroy pants and green tennis shoes, right? Right! We'd choose perhaps a tan pair of slim pants and a tan turtleneck sweater and simple slip-on shoes in a shade darker than her tan clothes. That's a very clean and quiet look. (However, that colorful, youthful outfit that we joked about for Sally might be perfect on Margaret whose style words include girlie and vibrant.)

This is how everyone looks different from everyone else. There are no cookie cutter recipes here. You have your own individual recipe and your way of putting it together will be unique.

This is all very important when we start building outfits. If "feminine" is one of your style words, then I'm interested in knowing what's in your closet already that says *feminine*. If there's nothing in your closet to work with that's feminine, do you know what you need?

I've created a Glossary of Style Words that is to help you detail how to achieve the look of your style recipe. I trust with all the work you've done honing your style words — cutting out pictures, putting them in your binder — that you have a pretty good idea how you would dress for your style recipe. Often images of outfits show up in women's minds like a slide show as soon as they have identified the style words that resonate for them. In case there are areas that are less than clear for you, the glossary will help give you a picture of how to express a specific style word in your recipe. For instance, if dramatic is a style word in your recipe, look up "Dramatic" in the style glossary that follows and discover *7* things:

1. AKA: "Also knows as" these similar style words

2. The overall "look"

3. What a casual outfit would look like

4. What a dressier outfit would look like

5. Key colors, textures, and patterns you'd expect to choose from

6. Hair and makeup that would suit that style word

7. Five key pieces that could be in a wardrobe

Look through the glossary for more ideas on how to dress in keeping with your style words. See if more words resonate with you and want to be added to your recipe. Grab a highlighter and mark the words you're attracted to and that represent some things you absolutely want to try.

GLOSSARY OF STYLE WORDS

ADORABLE

AKA: girlie, youthful, cute, sweet, lively, charming

THE LOOK: somewhat childlike, cute and innocent, playful and active, put together thoughtfully but look free and happy

A CASUAL OUTFIT: red and white plaid pedal pushers, white cotton tee, white flip-flops with cherries on them, red-and-white small beaded necklace, cropped jean jacket

A DRESSIER OUTFIT: bias cut knee-length plaid skirt, fitted tank top, cardigan over the tank with round crystal buttons, Mary Jane shoes

KEY COLORS, TEXTURES AND PATTERNS: pink, baby blue, yellow, bright pastels; no shiny fabrics; small to medium prints

HAIR AND MAKEUP: hair in pigtails with barrettes and bright-colored ponytail holders, a natural glowing face with lip gloss and mascara

FIVE KEY PIECES: pink tank top with daisies across the neckline, floral small handbag, bright-colored flip flops, loose jeans cuffed at the bottom, cropped cardigan with kitty cat buttons

SO ADORABLE
Pink, baby blue, hair in pigtails, a natural glowing face that everyone just wants to pinch?

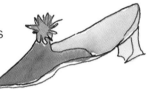

CLASSIC

AKA: intelligent, regal, conservative, traditional

THE LOOK: simple, understated, doesn't change much from year-to-year, nothing is body hugging, no frilly clothes

A CASUAL OUTFIT: khaki pleated pant, crisp white shirt with navy cardigan draped over the shoulders, navy sneakers, brown woven belt, brown shoulder bag

A DRESSIER OUTFIT: black straight-legged wool slacks, ivory cashmere twin-set with pearl buttons, Hermes or look-alike scarf over the shoulders, pearls, thin watch, fine leather belt, and Ferragamo-type pumps

KEY COLORS, TEXTURES AND PATTERNS: navy blue, camel, white, black, wine; mostly smooth and crisp textures with some tweeds; plaids, stripes and pinstripes, small polka dots

HAIR AND MAKEUP: pageboy cut, very neat; no trends in makeup, an even face — no one feature is highlighted strongly
FIVE KEY PIECES: cardigan set, pearls, basic black suit (with a lapeled jacket and pleated pant and knee-length straight skirt), thin Cartier-style watch, cableknit sweater

CREATIVE

AKA: arty, cutting edge, interesting, shows flair, unique, quirky, imaginative, unconventional, innovative

THE LOOK: very original ensembles, putting unusual pieces together that come from varied sources like vintage stores, garage sales and discount stores as well as designer racks; one print with the rest of the outfit in solids and a large colorful necklace, or in the winter, colorful scarves wrapped two times around the neck, making a thick collar

A CASUAL OUTFIT: green pants, a butter-colored shirt with a great orange handbag that screams "energy" and orange loafers that match

A DRESSIER OUTFIT: bias-cut hand-dyed tea length dress with painted jacket that blends with the dress, a multicolor beaded necklace, metallic and beaded sandals

KEY COLORS, TEXTURES, AND PATTERNS: all colors are possible choices, particularly creating unexpected color combinations, also black and dark tones; textures are also mixed together — smooth and shiny with furry and nappy, sheer textures; prints can be plaid or bold florals, or both together, strong graphic patterns, asymmetrical patterns, paisley, abstracts

HAIR AND MAKEUP: a lot of variety exists from short and spiky hair to long hair pulled up and twisted and held back with ribbons or barrettes or bleached white hair with red tips or black hair with blue highlights; a lot of emphasis in makeup is on a feature such as dark smoky eyes or bright red lips

FIVE KEY PIECES: artist's original pieces like a painted coat, MOMA (Museum of Modern Art) jewelry pieces, woven leather hobo bag, patchwork cowboy boots

THE CREATIVE TYPE
Do you often put together very one-of-a-kind outfits that no one could assemble but you?

DRAMATIC

AKA: striking, powerful, stunning, sophisticated, daring

THE LOOK: very strong, defined design lines in clothing, strong focal point either in the face or a portion of the body, something in the ensemble is isolated and holds your attention

A CASUAL OUTFIT: black poly/spandex cropped pants, bright red sleeveless top, red mules, ruby earrings (studs)

A DRESSIER OUTFIT: black tube dress with thick magenta stripe down the center, black shoes with magenta detail, magenta scarf wrapped around neck with the tails going down the back of the dress

KEY COLORS, TEXTURES, AND PATTERNS: bright red, eggplant, Kelly green, magenta, lemon yellow, black and white; shimmery textures, attention-grabbing textures whether it's fur, fabric with metallic threads running through it, or something with a rubberized surface; bold graphic prints, large scale patterns, animal prints

HAIR AND MAKEUP: big and/or unnaturally red hair, chin-length hair gelled close to the head or pulled tight into a bun; bright red lipstick, kohl eyeliner

FIVE KEY PIECES: show-stopper unique pieces that display a lot of workmanship like a Chinese embroidered knee-length coat, red leather pants, pointy black boots, velvet duster, red skirt suit (with a strong shoulder line and shiny black buttons)

DRAMA QUEEN
Do you love attention grabbing colors and textures—fur, metallic thread, bold prints?

ECLECTIC

AKA: original, interesting, unique, Bohemian, gypsy, innovative, off-beat, imaginative, playful

THE LOOK: mixes patterns, doesn't wear any logos, mixes vintage with new things, looks thrown together but actually is very well thought out and balanced, stylized accessories in exaggerated shapes, every item could be a stand-alone piece

A CASUAL OUTFIT: pink jeans, lime-green fuzzy sweater, leopard boot, stretchy leopard gloves

A DRESSIER OUTFIT: a slip as a dress, rhinestone shoes, a shimmery scarf with jeweled tassels as a shawl

KEY COLORS, TEXTURES, AND PATTERNS: all colors, mixed together, any texture mixed together, multiple patterns worn together but balanced, patterns that could be in upholstery fabrics
HAIR AND MAKEUP: hair dyed blond with roots showing; or blue, red, or green streaks in hair; bright lipstick, bright eye shadow with multiple colors used, runway model makeup
FIVE KEY PIECES: lunch box as a purse, antique kimono (made into a dress), red square-rimmed glasses, patchwork coat, purple velvet broad brimmed floppy hat

ELEGANT

ECLECTIC OR ELEGANT Which would you choose – a lime green fuzzy sweater or an emerald green silk shirt?

AKA: clear, rich, simple, sophisticated, luxurious, classy, quiet, refined
THE LOOK: straight, uncluttered style lines, lean on details, fabrics look luxurious and expensive
A CASUAL OUTFIT: gunmetal gray cashmere sweat pants with a matching hooded pullover sweatshirt, ballet flats, small charcoal leather backpack
A DRESSIER OUTFIT: champagne colored flowing satin pajama-style pants with a matching fine cashmere tunic top, pearlized sandals, simple pearl necklace and earrings
KEY COLORS, TEXTURES, AND PATTERNS: charcoal, taupe, ivory, black, burgundy, one single color worn head-to-toe; shiny, smooth fabrics like satin and silk charmeuse, fine knits that are smooth; very few patterns except for jacquards or other subtly woven fabrics that create a pattern
HAIR AND MAKEUP: straight hair or a French twist or long loose curls, hair is shiny and clean; a natural face but polished, smooth even skin tone
FIVE KEY PIECES: pearl necklace, ivory cashmere turtleneck sweater, sheath dress and matching jacket, diamond posts, signature handbag

FEMININE

AKA: delicate, pretty, soft, womanly
THE LOOK: clothes show the female shape, shoes show

the toes, heels, or ankles; a soft overall look, graceful lines, no hard edges or sharp angles in the silhouette

A CASUAL OUTFIT: A flowing pastel blue floral print skirt with an ivory blouse that has small pleats or tucks, strappy sandals, a straw hat with a wide brim, glass beaded necklace

A DRESSIER OUTFIT: apricot long silk dress with a ruffled hem, clear Lucite-heeled sandals, Swarovski crystal drop earrings, beaded clutch evening bag

KEY COLORS, TEXTURES, AND PATTERNS: neutrals as in cream, champagne, blush pink, soft pastels including soft aqua, French blue, light yellow; fine textures; prints are delicate-to-medium scale floral prints

HAIR AND MAKEUP: soft pink lips and nail polish, subtle makeup colors

FIVE KEY PIECES: ivory lace blouse, sheer slip dress, pink suede jacket, open-toed sandals, cardigan sweater with pearl buttons and fur trim

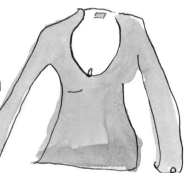

HIPPIE
**Flowing skirts,
sandals, denim,
fringes, layered
clothing?**

HIPPIE

AKA: earth mother, goddess

THE LOOK: loose-fitting, layered clothes with an emphasis on accessories such as fringed shawls, low-slung belts, beaded jewelry; clothes look worn in

A CASUAL OUTFIT: flair jeans slung low on hips, peasant blouse, Birkenstocks, shell and leather fringed belt

A DRESSIER OUTFIT: long empire-waist dark floral dress, purple velvet long coat, beaded choker at the neck, fringed tall suede boots

KEY COLORS, TEXTURES, AND PATTERNS: denim, muted colors with some jewel tones in velvets or corduroys; tweedy textures, corduroy, suede and distressed leather; paisley, florals, stripes, lace — lots of things mixed together

HAIR AND MAKEUP: long, wavy hair, flowing hair or braided hair; no makeup, or if wearing makeup, it looks all natural, lip balm

FIVE KEY PIECES: Birkenstock sandals, flowing prairie skirt, hemp choker, embellished jeans, big fringed suede shoulder bag

MYSTERIOUS

AKA: solitary, private, subtle, goddess, unconventional, serious

THE LOOK: a Tarot reader look; overall dark clothing with accents that include long, sheer scarves embellished with velvet and mirrors; all black clothing with mixed textures, sometimes heavy boots contrasting with the flowing fabrics

A CASUAL OUTFIT: black velour skirt and tunic, fringed metallic scarf around the neck, soft black flat boots, silver bangles, hoop earrings

A DRESSIER OUTFIT: velvet pants, velvet tunic with rich satin lining, lace-up heeled boots, lots of bangles, crystal beads at the neck, a head wrap

KEY COLORS, TEXTURES, AND PATTERNS: black, muddy blackened versions of colors

HAIR AND MAKEUP: long, loose hair with parts pulled back, unusual color added to tips; smoky eyes, bright or pale mouth

FIVE KEY PIECES: black lace-up boots, scarves with mirrors on them, hoop earrings, slouch velvet shoulder bag, black velvet slouchy coat

MYSTERY GIRL
**Boots, bangles,
smoky eyes,
scarves—do you
like to have an
air of mystery?**

NATURAL

AKA: earthy, relaxed, laid back, leisurely, comfortable, warm, approachable, nurturing, casual

THE LOOK: loose-fitting, 100 percent cotton sweatpants with elastic waistband (nothing is constricting), no synthetic clothing, clothes are made in the USA (no sweatshop labor), emphasis is on comfort, natural fibers and easy fit

A CASUAL OUTFIT: tan cargo pant, brown suede shirt-jacket, cream ribbed tee, clogs

A DRESSIER OUTFIT: suede tan A-line skirt, chunky ivory turtle neck sweater, tan riding boots, turquoise and silver jewelry

KEY COLORS, TEXTURES, AND PATTERNS: sand, oatmeal, khaki, brown, sage green, rust; open, loose weaves, medium to rough (nubby) textures in cotton, linen, rayon, Tencel, flannel; plaids, tweeds, stripes, checks

HAIR AND MAKEUP: short to long hair in easy care styles; coconut lip balm
FIVE KEY PIECES: shell necklace, cotton-twill barn jacket with red-plaid flannel lining, cotton crew neck tees, blue jeans, flannel shirt

SENSUAL

AKA: refined, sophisticated, rich, soft
THE LOOK: a sensual woman looks like her only worry is picking out her toenail polish color, all pieces are yummy to the touch whether wrapped in a cashmere shawl or a cashmere sweatsuit
A CASUAL OUTFIT: sheer soft blouse with ruffles at the cuffs over a thin tank top, low slung drapey drawstring pants, ballet flats
A DRESSIER OUTFIT: jersey knit, slinky long dress, open-toed sandals, crocheted shawl with long fringe, drop earrings
KEY COLORS, TEXTURES, AND PATTERNS: taupe, ivory, dusty blues and greens, violet, yellow, winter white, midnight navy, oyster, bone, taupe; fine textures in fabrics like cashmere, Egyptian cotton, Irish linen, tropical weight wools; lustrous fluid fabrics like silk charmeuse; refined patterns, lots of solids
HAIR AND MAKEUP: soft, easy hair styles, long to short, tousled; dewy skin, wet looking lips, soft neutral eye makeup
FIVE KEY PIECES: cashmere hooded, close-fitting sweatshirt, velvet pants, oversized shawl in which you can wrap yourself, cashmere or a sheer silk, jersey knit skirt and T-shirt top, bathrobe style cashmere coat

SEXY GIRL
Soft, slinky, seductive. Do these words describe you and your clothes?

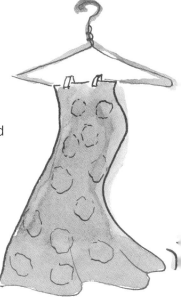

SEXY

AKA: alluring, seductive, passionate, exciting, vivacious, diva
THE LOOK: attention-getting in close-fitting, body-conscious silhouettes as well as eye-catching fabrics that shine or dazzle
A CASUAL OUTFIT: slim-fitting jeans, wide V-neck red jersey-knit short-sleeved tee, red-heeled mules, slim hoop earrings with beads dangling from them
A DRESSIER OUTFIT: strapless body-hugging red dress with lots of Lycra in it, strappy heels that wrap up past the ankle

KEY COLORS, TEXTURES, AND PATTERNS: red, black; shiny and shimmery smooth textures, generous doses of leather, suede, and fur, beaded fabrics; animal prints

HAIR AND MAKEUP: hair can be short and tousled looking or long and wavy; smoky eyes, nude lips with gloss or red lips, strong emphasis on eyes or mouth

FIVE KEY PIECES: off-the-shoulder black-knit top, beaded sleeveless top, slim cigarette pants, open-toed sandaled heels

SPORTY

AKA: athletic, active, natural, playful

THE LOOK: body-hugging clothing with a high spandex content, cotton-and-Lycra blend separates, street clothes are modified versions of the sport versions

A CASUAL OUTFIT: elastic-waist loose Capri pants with stripes down the side, sports bra tank top, sports watch, backless athletic shoes, hooded sweatshirt, sports cap

A DRESSIER OUTFIT: short cotton tank dress, leather flip-flops with terrain bottoms, sweater wrapped around the waist, 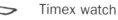 Timex watch

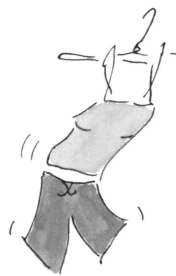

KEY COLORS, TEXTURES, AND PATTERNS: bright colors or natural tones, navy blue, black, white; smooth textures in tech fabrics; racer stripes, color blocking (side panels contrast with front and back panels of a jersey top)

HAIR AND MAKEUP: ponytail; waterproof mascara, sunscreen face lotion, cherry chapstick

FIVE KEY PIECES: fitted hooded sweatshirt, white halter tee with built-in bra, tennies in every color, short denim skirt, colorful windbreakers

URBAN

AKA: hip-hop culture

THE LOOK: rugged, industrial looking, rough, everything's heavy duty, faded T-shirts, worn leather jacket, nothing looks brand-new

A CASUAL OUTFIT: baggy, low-slung khakis, Pumas or Adidas, body-hugging tank

A DRESSIER OUTFIT: black patent-leather short skirt, black lace top (see-through) with corset underneath, hoop earrings with rhinestones

KEY COLORS, TEXTURES, AND PATTERNS: dirty denim, black, metal colors, white, khaki, black on black; rough textures, stretch mesh; camouflage patterns

HAIR AND MAKEUP: hair in mini braids, corn rows or tousled up on head with bobby pins, or hair is dyed in an edgy color, hair has something unusual going on with it; dark heavy eyes, maroon lips

FIVE KEY PIECES: heavy-duty belt with grommets, worn leather jacket, baggy jean style pants, Pumas

SPORTY TYPE
Can you always
be found in active,
athletic looks?

Mixing It Up

If you are like most people, you are a combination of characteristics. You may be both arty and conservative, or sexy and earthy. You might exude three or four different characteristics. Because most of us are a combination of one type or another, here are three examples of how to combine characteristics.

Arty Conservative: Trim navy blue suit, crisp white shirt and far out shoes (Manola Blahniks or another type of shoe that looks like a museum piece). Add a really artistic, creative pin that you picked up at the Museum of Modern Art plus a really whackadoodle haircut (think "rock star") with minimal makeup. The suit and shirt are conservative as well as the color, but the accessory (either the pin on the suit lapel or the shoes) is arty and something on the face is arty, in this case, the haircut.

Elegant Playful: Black fine-knit turtleneck with matching straight-legged flowing pants (both the color and the simplicity of these two pieces are elegant). Add a lunchbox style handbag with superhero action figures on it in multiple colors, lipstick red ankle boots that pick up one of the colors in the lunchbox handbag. Red lipstick pulls the red up to the face. Hair is pulled back in a tight ponytail that moves easily. The movement of the ponytail is playful as is the novel handbag. The red accents in the boots and lipstick add spark and fun.

Sophisticated Hippie: Black velvet skirt and matching cowl-neck pullover tee with an American Indian conch belt slung low on the hip, tall black riding boots, large fringed suede shoulder bag, silver bangles stacked up the arm, hoop earrings. The shoulder bag could be in a fine leather (more expensive than the one you bought in your freshman year in college) but have the natural flow of a hippie styled bag. The belt could also be more on the sophisticated side, a cleaner design. The riding boots fit the feel of the outfit but still blend sleekly with the clothes. Creating a clean, uncluttered line is sophistication.

MAKE A STYLE SHRINE:

Go through your closet and pull three clothing or jewelry items that are the strongest representations of looks you love. If you have a wild side to you, it may be your python print pants. If you are a true romantic, it might be a lacy handkerchief. Put these items together as a strong visual reminder of parts of you that are essential to representing your style. Throw them over a chair or make an altar. Did you find any NEW style words or recipes you just can't wait to try? Write them here while they are fresh in your mind.

MY NEW STYLE WORDS:

_____

_____

_____

_____

_____

Now that you have all your New Style Words written down, tinker with them. Look at them for a few days in a row. Do they still **resonate?** Every single word? If one or two words were just a passing fancy and don't "zing" past day two, consider how important they really are to you. Toss them if they don't feel right. Keep this list current and honest. That's how it energizes and serves you. Keep these words in your binder along with your collages. Put a copy in your wallet for when you're shopping. Pull out the list and put the items you're considering to buy to the test. Are they in alignment? Along with your pictures, your style words are another guide for getting the look you want with

the clothes you LOVE.

The Interview

I BET YOU'RE JUST ITCHING to start working with your clothes. All this talk about past experiences has created a palette of fresh ideas that you're aching to work with. Shopping stories — yours as well as others — have you salivating to shop. Taking a look at your attributes and what you want to focus on (your eye color, your shapely legs, your ebony hair) has you anxious to get out there and highlight them with a new blouse (in one of your best colors) a belt, or a slim pant. You can't wait to play with your style recipe and you're so ready to be out of your ruts and doing something new that your imagination is running wild with ideas. So you know what? If you feel like you want to go shopping, do it. You've done some superb work already. You deserve an outing. This won't be your super duper shopping trip that pulls your whole wardrobe together. We're not quite there yet. I have a few more questions to ask you and then of course, a visit to your closet is in order. But for now, let's celebrate! You're halfway there.

I've got a few ideas for you. Take a look at them and choose what you'd like to do to honor your good work so far. And then, when you're refreshed, start the interview process where you'll look specifically at your current wardrobe and make some plans to move it toward that wardrobe I promised you — the one that works 100%, 100% of the time. But hey, that's for later. Indulge yourself now in some

fun, fun, fun!

We're-Halfway-There Treats

1. **Attack a rut.** Pick out one of your ruts and go shopping for something that will get you far, far away from that rut. If you have a buddy, the two of you can go shopping together, supporting each other to counter your ruts with a creative new idea. If you absolutely fall in love with something you find (remember, Do the Love Thing!) buy it. *I trust you.* However, I do suggest you shop at a store that has a generous return policy so you can take it back if you get it home and it doesn't look far enough away from your identified rut after all. Some ruts are hard to get away from and you might journey out once or twice before you get some new results. Keep the receipt handy and review your "rut buster" when you start building outfits so you can be sure it fits in with your style words and wardrobe priorities.

2. **Practice a few fashion strategies only in a non-clothing arena —** do it with food! Go to a restaurant you've been really wanting to go to (maybe with your buddy) and order exactly what you want from the menu. This gives you practice in doing the love thing, remembering that you're worth full price and not saving good things for good (like the fact that you're eating at this restaurant for no reason other than you want to!), good is right now! Use this relaxing time to catch up with yourself. Think back at where you started in this process and where you've come. Chat about it with your buddy or maybe a friend who has joined you for this mid-way celebration. And don't forget to look at the dessert menu!

3. **Play around in your closet and see if you can assemble outfits that match words from your style recipe.** Look through the style glossary and see if a craving for a specific item popped up when you read the listings for a casual outfit, dressy outfit or one of the five key pieces. If you don't have it, go out and satisfy that craving — just one or two items though! Coming up soon is plenty of opportunity for some serious shopping. So go out and buy that pair of tennis shoes in a fun color, or a bustier, or a shawl, or a pair of dangling earrings. You deserve it!

4. **March down to a makeup counter and play with makeup looks that go with your style recipe.** A terrific way to celebrate your progress is to experiment with your makeup colors, techniques or tools. Go to a

makeup counter and give the makeup person a few of your style words and see how this professional person interprets those words. She may have just the right shade of lipstick for a "dramatic" mouth or ideas for eye makeup for a "sensual" or "sexy" look. Don't feel like you have to buy the whole look when you're done. Maybe just a lipstick, blush or eye shadow color will do for now. Have fun!

Pick Up Your Pencils

Feel better now? I hope you had a great time and now are ready to sit down for the interview. Get ready for an interview that will focus on the most fascinating person in the world — YOU! These are the same questions I ask my clients. Your thoughtful answers will clarify what your current clothing needs are, what parts of your wardrobe you'll focus on first, what you're already doing that's really right and worth repeating. You'll get a chance to remind yourself of what you're moving away from and what you're moving toward in terms of how you express yourself in clothes. **There are still some gems to harvest** that will make your trip through your closet and your first shopping expedition both efficient and successful.

A comment about repetition: If you find that some answers overlap, that's all right. Sometimes it might seem that I'm asking you questions from slightly different angles. I am! It's as though I'm holding out a butterfly net and capturing as much information as I can so we can be really clear about your next steps. The work you do here will make the next steps easier for you. Some answers may sound similar. Good. You're starting to see some patterns. Patterns reinforce where you need to focus. Remember, repetition is a good thing.

Read through the questions and see how much of this you'd like to do with your buddy. I can imagine you lying back in the comfort of your couch or against the pillows of your bed and letting someone else ask you the questions and take the notes. If you prefer to do this with a buddy, you can be the star and your buddy can be Barbara Walters and then switch roles. Otherwise you can do this on your own. *Here we go!*

Identify What Works

The first thing I want to ask you is what do you have in your wardrobe that already works? Let your "favorites" tell you. Do you have a skirt made out of a fabric whose feel you love? Does it drape the way you like, swish and make a sound you like? How about color? Does a certain color work for you when you want to relax? Do you have a favorite color that *makes you feel alive?* Make an inventory of your favorite items. List what it is that works so well for you. Then list the benefit you derive from it.

FOR EXAMPLE:

ITEM	WHAT I LOVE	WHY IT WORKS
Green suit	Monochromatic colors	I look tall and thin; sleek, high fashion
Gold watch	It's elegant and dressy	Makes me feel polished

WHAT WORKS FOR YOU:

ITEM	WHAT I LOVE	WHY IT WORKS

Envy is just wishing for what you think you can't have —and guess what, you CAN have it.

Dream Shopping

Start a dream shopping list. This is a list that expands on what you already know works. Maybe you listed comfort, fit, color, texture, style. These are your "must haves." They are the target in your satisfaction zone.

So you **love** a winter jacket you own. Want to consider a similar one for summer? So you **love** the fit of those black pants. Have you thought of getting them in red?

If you could fill your closet with what you love and what works, what would be there? You may want more texture, pattern, or color but not know the exact items they'd appear in. **That's okay.** Just write down the essence of what you want.

MY DREAM SHOPPING LIST

_____

_____

_____

_____

_____

_____

_____

Whom do you admire in terms of their looks or the way they have matched their personality to their looks?

Think of boyfriends. When they buy you your favorite flowers and you express your pleasure, they are likely to do it again. That's true of clothes too. If a neckline on a blouse makes you feel fabulous, the next time you see a top that mimics that neckline and it's in a color you love, you'll buy it, wear it, and be pleased all over again. **Repeating what works is good clothes sense.**

Identify a Fashion Heroine

Is there someone in your life whose style, look, or wardrobe you secretly covet? I encourage you to look at anyone you have envied in terms of their look and really think about what it is that you envy about them. It's okay to use envy as a guiding light right now. It's not something I normally encourage; however, envy is just wishing for what you think you can't have — and guess what, you can have it.

Is there someone in the arts, the media, the movies or the news whose style you admire? It's okay to borrow from the masters. During the Renaissance, that's what artists did. They painted replicas of fine art to see how it felt to execute at that level. I'm asking you to do the same kind of thing here. **Study the masters in your life and analyze what it is they do that you admire.**

Do you have a sister-in-law who looks put together without being showy? What is she doing? Do you have a friend who always delights you with the combinations of colors she dresses in? Write them down. Do you know someone who really has a signature look with her accessories? What is she doing?

One of my heroines is a woman who works at Saks Fifth Avenue in San Francisco. She often wears great-fitting pants and then adds tops that have a lot of interest in them. Either it's a T-shirt in a great print or a top with a lot of textural interest in the fabric, or the color provides a splashy contrast to the neutral pants. Since studying her, I've gotten bolder in my choices. When I go on automatic and come close to one of my ruts, I think about her and what she'd do. It keeps me on my toes, stretching my fashion legs.

Another fashion heroine of mine is my writing buddy, Christie. She has a beautiful collection of beaded necklaces that repeat whatever color she wears. She'll wear amber beads with a pumpkin blouse, or a smoky topaz necklace with a dusty sage-green top. Her jewelry always makes her outfit pop. I was never a necklace wearer but she changed my mind. I'm inspired by her, but I don't look like her. When I borrow from her "ideas," I translate them into MY design sense.

So go hunting for ideas on people you see. And make notes about them here.

LOOKS I LOVE ON OTHERS:

_____

_____

_____

_____

_____

_____

_____

94

TRY THIS:

Pore through the fashion/media magazines and look at actresses. Stylists are paid a lot of money to make them look great for their movie premieres. Steal some ideas. Do you find someone who has coloring like yours? See what she does with her makeup and the colors she's wearing. Some people really have an affinity for a certain actress's look. See what she's up to. Realize that there are lots of bad looks out there and some actresses specialize in them. Just look for what wildly attracts you. You may see a combination of a dress and a certain shoe style that inspires you for this season — or a casual at-home look that you would like to steal and use for yourself. Spend an hour or so looking through magazines and then write down in your binder some of your favorite looks, ones you'd like to try.

What Do You Want Your Clothes to Say about You?

Clothes speak for you. When you haven't opened your mouth, your clothes have already said a whole bunch about you. You can choose what they say. What qualities do you want to project when you walk into a room? What do you want people to be thinking?

EXAMPLE: *"There's Mary, she is so brilliant."*

"There's _____ (your name). She is so _____ (qualities).

> Before you even open your mouth, your clothes have said a lot about you. What are they saying? Is it what you want to hear?

Now pick some descriptive words like the following: put-together, bright, approachable, funny, cute, sensitive, deep, expressive, creative, soulful, spiritual, understated. Got it?

What would you like others to see in you? Maybe what you want others to know about you in your professional life is different than in your personal life. Susan may want to emphasis her efficiency and strong work ethic at the office, but would like to let people know she's lots of fun at a party. She makes distinctions between her personal and her professional life.

If it suits you better, make two (or more) lists to reflect the qualities you want to be known for in different areas of your life.

LIST THOSE QUALITIES NOW:

_____

_____

_____

_____

TRY THIS:

As you describe what you'd like others to say about you, think about how you have walked into a room lately. If that ideal image isn't 100 percent, what percentage would you say you are at right now? Are you 80 percent of your ideal image? 50 percent there? 25 percent there? What can you see right now that you could do to bring you closer to 100 percent?

Knowing

What do people "get" about you right away? There are things about you that people just know instantly. You barely have to open your mouth and people know this about you — that you are vivacious or bright or kind or outrageous. What things about you do you think are apparent right away?

LIST THEM:

_____

_____

_____

_____

If you have any doubts about these things, ask your buddy to give you some feedback.

Wishing

Okay, now think about those things that people don't know about you. *What wouldn't you mind sharing?* In fact, what do you want people to know about you? Maybe you are very earnest and serious, and you wish people would see your witty side. Or you're really kind and patient, but you wish people would see your irreverence. Maybe you are the frisky life-of-the-party person, but you'd like people to have a clue about how respected you are in your profession.

What little known parts of you do you want people to know now?

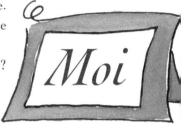

LIST THEM:

_____

_____

_____

_____

_____

A BUDDY EXERCISE:

Get with your buddy (or a team of buddies) and brainstorm how to bring inside "qualities" to the outside. Think of this as a game. The goal is to match inside qualities to your outsides through clothing choices. For instance, Sue wanted to be known for her quiet elegance. Her friend knew a banker who had a look that could be identified that way. The banker wore solid colors head to toe in soothing colors-all ivory in a blouse and skirt in the same fabric, or all sage green in a tunic top over non-creased straight legged pants. She was soothing to look at, and that's what Sue wanted.

An artist I admire always wears loose flowered shirts and low top tennis shoes in one of the bright colors of the shirt. It's easy to think of her as an artist because her clothes are bold, vibrant, creative and unusual.

The quality Helen wanted to demonstrate in her clothes was luxury. Carolyn had an aunt who was an image of luxury. This aunt never left the house without makeup, a matching suit, stockings, and pumps. Although that look was too formal for Helen, she could translate the information to fit her own casual lifestyle.

Now that you have some examples to work from, get some brainstorming going. Throw out a quality and see what vivid pictures come up. Have fun!

Moving Away From, Moving Toward

In order to get somewhere, you need to know where you're starting from and where you're headed. If you're headed to Tennessee, you have a great chance of getting there if you know you're starting from Minnesota. It's the same with clothes.

In order to get somewhere you haven't been before in clothes, you need to nail down where you're starting from and identify where you're headed. The *place to start* is to tell the truth (without judgment) about what's been going on with you and clothes. Then identify what you'd like to have going on. Think about your style, your closet, getting dressed, your choices, the variety of things to choose from, the money you spend, the time you spend. What's not working? What frustrates you? What bugs you? Those are things you are moving away from.

Now, if the problems or issues were gone, what would you like to have replace them? That's what you're moving towards. Look deeply and honestly and then think expansively about what you want. What you want can absolutely come true, but you need to identify where you have been and where you want to go in order for change to weave its magic and transform your life. Your dreams depend on you to identify them. Here are some examples.

By telling the truth about what you want to become, you can let go of ways that have hindered you from expressing this more.

MOVING AWAY FROM:	MOVING TOWARD:
confusion	confidence
lack of focus	consistency
playing it safe	being okay with being smart, sassy, lovely, "in your face"
being all over the place	a distinctive look and style
unsure	more accurately reflecting who I am
being invisible	being powerful
wearing a small # of clothes	wearing everything in my closet
looking tired, boring	looking vivacious and happy

MOVING AWAY FROM: MOVING TOWARD:

_____   _____

_____   _____

_____   _____

_____   _____

MOVING AWAY FROM: MOVING TOWARD:

_____   _____

_____   _____

_____   _____

_____   _____

Okay, you've told the **truth.** Now it's easier to let go because you've created a map to where you're heading. (There's that Tell-the-Truth-Let-Go-Create mantra again, helping you along!) Let your intuitive side help create a new response to your old patterns. When you're out shopping and you're looking at the same ordinary white blouse that you always buy, remember you are moving away from ordinary and moving toward **extraordinary.** Put that ordinary blouse down and keep looking for the extraordinary one. It's there for you!

BUDDY EXERCISE:

Have a buddy talk. It helps to tell someone where you've been and where you're headed. By letting go, you create space for better things to come in and satisfy you. If you are moving away from hanging around home in raggedy sweats, then the easy next step is identifying what you'd rather hang out in. Once identified, it's easy to get that thing that you'd feel great in.

This is a great place to create a ritual. Write what you're moving away from on pieces of paper and then read them to your buddy. Say a blessing for where you've been and then as a symbol of letting go, burn the pieces of paper. It's amazing how a simple act like this makes things happen more easily.

"I'm letting go and I'm moving forward" is your new battle cry. Talk with your buddy about what you're moving toward. And then switch and let her tell you what she's moving toward. Hearing other people's stories will reinforce your own resolve and give you momentum to take new action steps.

With your buddy's help, come up with five action steps to move you closer to where you want to be. Can you just feel the changes coming? You're on your way. Thank your buddy for being such a great help.

MY ACTION STEPS:

1.
2.
3.
4.
5.

I Used to _____, but Now I _____.

Now I'm interested in your current life — the one right here. Not the life you lived last year or five years ago. That's history. It's good to know what you're moving away from and what you're moving toward. It's even better to see where that shows up specifically in your life. Let's continue separating your past from the present with an "I used to _____, but now I _____." exercise. By reviewing in detail what "was" true for you, we can get closer to what "is" true for you now.

CHECK OUT THESE EXAMPLES:

I used to need lots of variety, but now having fewer things feels better.

I used to want classic clothes, but now I want to add some trendy things to my wardrobe.

I used to love the color orange, but now I'm crazy about blues.

I used to focus my wardrobe on work clothes, but now I want to focus on date clothes.

I used to not care how I looked, but now it matters to me.

NOW IT'S YOUR TURN:

I used to _____,

but now I _____.

I used to _____,

but now I _____.

I used to _____,

but now I _____.

I used to _____,

but now I _____.

ARE YOU SEEING SOME FRESH NEEDS?
WRITE OUT YOUR OBSERVATIONS HERE:

_____

_____

_____

_____

_____

_____

_____

Clothes for Your Lifestyle

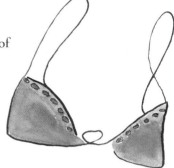

What do you need clothes for? Think about all the parts of your life. What are your **roles**? Are you a student, mother, wife, partner, employee, employer, volunteer, auntie, grandmother, head of a service board at the local theater company, athlete, traveler? Each role involves activities that require clothes. Sometimes one role involves a few activities that require changes of clothes. For instance, Susan works for a non-profit organization. She works in an office that is casual. She also makes presentations to businesses during luncheons, which requires more professional attire. Her role is "work." Her activities include working in the office, making presentations, representing the organization at networking events. Another role is being a mom to her ten and eleven-year-old daughters. Her **activities** include going to their softball and basketball games, hanging out with them at home, driving them places, taking them shopping, etc. In her role as "friend," she goes out to dinner and to movies, attends book group, goes to coffee shops for chats.

Take a minute now and list the roles in your life and the activities that go along with them.

ROLES AND ACTIVITIES:

ROLES   ACTIVITIES

_____   _____

                                    _____

                                    _____

_____   _____

                                    _____

                                    _____

ROLES		ACTIVITIES

ROLE:
Community
Volunteer
ACTIVITIES:
Staff phone lines
Attend fund-raisers
Direct meetings

Clothes for All Reasons

Think of things you do in your social, personal, work, public and family life. Do you need clothes for work, dates, exercising, playing, gardening, volunteering, going to church, to school, traveling, attending board meetings, going to dinner parties, movies, clubs?

You need clothes for the whole of your life. That includes sleeping and relaxing too. We're not just focusing on one part of your wardrobe, although you may be tackling these things one-at-a-time, making priorities. The clothes you hang out in at home are just as important as the ones you wear to church. Every part of your life matters to me. Our job isn't done until we address every situation in which you wear clothes.

When you look into a crystal ball, are there things coming up in your future that will require new clothes? Getting into a new sport? Planning a trip to a place where the climate is different? What's out there? Include it all.

Look through the following list and **assess your wardrobe.** Are you satisfied, does an area need improvement or a complete overhaul? Check it now.

CATEGORY:	OK	NEEDS WORK	NEEDS OVERHAUL
Work	☐	☐	☐
Date	☐	☐	☐
Religious Services	☐	☐	☐
Home	☐	☐	☐
Sports	☐	☐	☐
Sports Events	☐	☐	☐
Casual Parties	☐	☐	☐
Dressy Parties	☐	☐	☐
Formal Parties	☐	☐	☐
Weddings	☐	☐	☐
Funerals	☐	☐	☐
Baptisims	☐	☐	☐
Bar/Bat Mitzvahs	☐	☐	☐
Bedroom Clothes	☐	☐	☐
Sleeping Clothes	☐	☐	☐
Gardening	☐	☐	☐
Camping	☐	☐	☐

What I Need and Want from My Clothes

Clothes are like puppy dogs. They just want to please the heck out of you. They can be as responsive as the kindest friend you ever had. You just need to tell them what you want and what you need.

That's what you're going to do now. You may find yourself repeating some things you've already "sorta" said somewhere else. That's okay. The more often and the louder you hear it coming from yourself, the more likely you'll move towards honoring your needs and wants. Your desires may have been buried for a long time so recognizing them may be a bit of a project. Don't worry, you're getting there!

Watch your
wardrobe shape
 itself to be
what you want and
need. By putting
your thoughts in
order, you'll give
your clothes a
chance to
follow suit.

This is like sitting down to *make the list* of what you'd like in your dream house. Or it's the list of qualities you want in a mate. I'll bet you've made lists like that before. If you just accept anything that comes along without thinking about it, chances are it's not going to be what you really want. It doesn't matter whether that's a house, a relationship, or a wardrobe.

Here are some ways people have responded to this exercise. They want clothes that are comfortable, clothes that are unique to match their personalities. They want to look put together, to not follow the latest trends. They need clothes to help them feel professional in their jobs, to help them feel more sexy, to stand out, to show they care about themselves.

Make a list of all the things you can think of that you'd like from your clothes.

WHAT I WANT & NEED FROM MY CLOTHES:

_____

_____

_____

_____

_____

TRY THIS:
Get rid of what's in the way of your caring wardrobe. Okay, let's just do a little thinking right here. If you want your clothes to be more comfortable, then what is in your closet right now that you never put on because it's too uncomfortable? Maybe your too-tight jeans. Or that skirt with a waistband that is stiff. Go to your closet and pull out those things that don't give you what you want from your wardrobe.

Wrap It up

I asked you to look at your life and see what clothes you need for all your activities. What are your big "aha's"? Where don't you have anything to wear? I bet it's starting to make sense to you where the holes are and where your wardrobe isn't taking care of you. Share this information with your buddy so when you go shopping, she can help you stay on track. Even though on paper we know we need dressy casual outfits, we may still gravitate to the workout section because we're comfortable shopping there. Your buddy can help you stay on track if she is privy to your needs.

Now that you've taken a close look at your own needs, wants and desires, identify the areas where you want to work first. Maybe one great outfit for each area of your life would feel like the place to start. Maybe parts of your wardrobe are abundant while others are deprived. What area requires your most urgent attention? Write in your priorities here.

MY PRIORITIES:

_____

_____

_____

_____

It's great to have copies of your interview answers in your binder. Put them in a section with a divider labeled "Interview" or "Assessments." You've been assessing your wardrobe and now you have the plans you need to create the wardrobe you've always wanted. Listening to yourself will reap you great rewards.

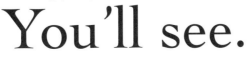

You'll see.

Closet Resolve

GET OUT YOUR CAMERA and go take a picture of your closet, right now, with the doors open. I'm serious. This is not to embarrass or shame you, this is to show you the "before" picture to compare with the "after" picture you'll take when we're finished. Believe me, you can't embarrass yourself around me. I've seen it all. I've been in more closets than you can imagine. Here are some things I find in a "typical" closet: a fifteen-year-old wedding dress, Christmas wrap, clothes that don't fit, clothes from college days and corporate office days, maternity clothes, vintage clothes, worn-out shoes, empty plastic dry-cleaning bags, yukky old fabric belts, self-tie belts from dresses long gone, roller skates, scarves falling off a hook, a shopping bag of gifts for upcoming family birthdays. And that's if she doesn't share a closet with her husband! In fact, there's so much stuff in there, it's a miracle that anyone gets dressed in the morning.

The Concept

Here's what I see for you. Opening that closet door just makes you happy. It's neat, organized, and pleasant to look at. Everything in there is your best friend. All the clothes are ready to wear. This means there are no hems falling, no buttons hanging, no ripped-open seams. The problems with any clothes have been repaired. *Everything fits!* Everything is in the current season. Out-of-season clothes are stored somewhere else. You can see your clothes and shoes. Putting outfits together is easy and creative.

What do you suppose the distance is between that closet and your closet now? Maybe a hundred miles? Let's close the gap. I'll provide the steps. You provide the time and energy. I might as well tell you right now, this is a project. But once you get the closet cleaned, you can add to the shopping list you started in the last chapter and then put outfits together that match your style words. That's just the beginning. The benefits of a cleaned-out closet are huge. Here are some comments my clients have made once they've done what you're about to do:

"I feel ten pounds lighter."

"This moved the stale energy out and now I want to clean my whole house."

"I actually feel more harmony among my family members."

"This gives me more time in the morning for sex."

Don't be surprised if your closet becomes a haven for you, a place where you just enjoy "being" because it's so calm and pleasant in there, like sitting on a bench in a Zen garden. Come on, let's make a trip to your closet feel like a trip to a health spa — rejuvenating and refreshing.

What to Expect

It is conceivable that you could accomplish all the phases of a closet clean-out in one big day, but don't push it. That is probably unrealistic for most of you. Two weekend dates in a row should take care of it with a few errands in between. See if you can manage that. Pacing and momentum are critical here. I know you have a life, a full life. By investing time now, you will enjoy that full life ten-fold and sooner than you think. In fact, your life will run so much more smoothly once you've worked through these phases, you'll be thrilled you made the effort.

This project takes some thought, preparation, and planning. Remember, you don't have to do it alone. You can enlist the help of a buddy or a team of buddies. You can farm your family out for the weekend or take a personal day from work. This is a job that takes time and will temporarily create chaos before it concludes with peace, order and satisfaction. I know lots about cleaning closets, so trust me. The more you pace yourself and complete each phase, the more momentum you'll have to tackle the next one. Celebrate in increments. Reward the

FOUND IN A TYPICAL CLOSET:

- Bridesmaid dress or two
- Family pictures in boxes
- Bicycle chain
- Empty shopping bags
- Yearbooks
- Tennis rackets

progress you make. If you get bogged down, take breaks. Review the personal assets section in Attitude Rehab or your binder. Reminding yourself of your gifts, talents, and resources is an energy booster. Your ordered closet will refresh you every day you get dressed.

Take five minutes, close your eyes, and visualize a closet that is everything you hope for. What's not working, doesn't fit, and is ancient history is gone and miles away. Think about the end of your big Closet Clean-out Day. Stare into your closet, all pristine, neat and orderly, clothes hanging that you are eager to wear, things you may actually have forgotten you had. You've let go of the albatross around your neck — a closet that was getting in the way of your life's working smoothly. How do you feel? Fantastic? Excellent! This is where you're headed.

Still got your eyes closed? Now think about how you're going to celebrate. Plan a fun reward. Champagne? A walking tour of your closet for your buddy, family, and neighborhood friends? A foot massage? A soak in the bathtub with bubbles? Tell me. You're going to do what? Great! I'm with you!

Phase I: Prep Work

I heard a statistic once that women wear one-tenth of the clothes in their closet. I'd have to say that's on the high side. So, look at your closet. Realize that probably 50 to 95 percent of it is going somewhere else, which could mean that a large volume of things will be moving out of your house. "Out" is the operative word in that last sentence. **Don't just move the stuff from room to room.** Expect to clear everything that isn't currently useful out of your space. Far away. Less is more, and don't forget, we will be adding things when you go shopping, so don't panic.

Planning the Export Strategy

Think about what you'll do with the clothes you weed out of your closet. Consignment stores take things in good shape, if they're current styles. Some stores are trendier than others so make some phone calls and find out. It's fun to get cash for things that don't work so you can reinvest in things that do. There are also charities. They take clothes and give you a tax deduction. Maybe you have relatives to give things to. Or maybe you'll follow my "Try This" exercise at the end of this chapter and plan a swap meet and invite your friends.

Realize ahead of time that what you're going to do with the things that are leaving your closet is a step you probably won't tackle the day of your closet clean-out. But don't lose momentum. Decide ahead of time where you're going to take things you no longer want. Find out their procedures for accepting donations before you arrive with bags in hand. It will save you time and hassle.

CONSIGNMENT STORE AND CHARITY POLICIES:

_____

_____

_____

_____

_____

_____

_____

Setting a Schedule

Okay, get out your calendar. Let's set some dates. Set your shopping date for gathering up your supplies and then set the date for your Closet Clean-out Day. I suggest the weekend. If both you and your buddy are doing this, alternate weekends for this project. Write down the date you plan to transfer all the clothes that are leaving your closet. How about a week to ten days after your clean-out day? Don't let that energy stall or stagnate.

Set a date when you'll have your alterations and repairs handled. Again, try to do this within the first week. Momentum is grace. Stay in the flow and this will be effortless.

Build in a day for fine-tuning everything within the week after your closet clean-out day. This is your date to get any containers you need that you didn't have when you cleaned out your closet. Often you have to get in there and move things around before you can see what kinds of storage units are going to work for you.

Plan a photo-shoot day, the day when everything is in picture perfect order in your closet. These are your "after" pictures. Oh, what fun! I can hardly wait to see them! This is also a good time to bring out the champagne and chocolates for you and your buddy.

STAY IN THE FLOW
Momentum is grace. Stay in the flow and this will be EFFORTLESS.

SET YOUR DATES:

Buying Supplies Day	_____
Closet Clean-out Day	_____

FOLLOW UP:

Clothes Giveaway Day	_____
Alterations & Repair Day	_____
Photo-Shoot Day	_____

Phase II: Gathering Supplies

The next step is to shop for your supplies. Here's what you need for your Closet Clean-Out Day:

1. Large trash bags or empty boxes

2. A full-length mirror (this is non-negotiable)

3. Great music

4. Your celebratory beverage of choice plus snacks for the day

5. Empty shopping bags

6. Storage containers you love

7. Souvenir box (something to store things you'll keep because of the sentimental value, although they no longer serve as actual wearable clothes)

8. Matching hangers

9. Portable clothes rack (optional)

Containing Your Clothes

Let's talk about storage containers. Storing "like" things together is a fabulous revelation. You can store things in bureaus or drawers, but the more visible, the better. It's so easy to put things inside a drawer and forget about them. Hanging storage "shelves" that are made out of nylon and can be attached to your closet pole with Velcro are practical and fun. See-through plastic boxes store shoes. Tie racks make great scarf racks. Canvas storage containers are good for storing "out-of-season" clothes. Have a ball checking out storage possibilities for your closet. Go online to places like IKEA.com or containerstore.com or call for a free catalog from Hold Everything (1-800-421 2264) for creative storage solutions.

Clean out your closet **BEFORE** you call in a closet designer. Fewer clothes equal freed-up space. I've ripped out closet systems that were too cumbersome. Most of you just need a closet clean-out, not a remodel. Remember, when you get that 50 to 95 percent of clothes you don't wear and all that other home paraphernalia out of there, you're going to have space galore. *So don't do anything rash* until we've done the clean-out. If the benefits of a closet remodel are apparent, that's when you'll know.

Once you've weeded things out, you may find the storage solutions you were going to use aren't really what you need after all. That's what "closet follow-up day" is for. Save your receipts so you can take things back and buy what serves you best. How you store things is just as personal as how you get dressed so use the same principles here as you do with your clothes. Buy what you love. Be delighted to reach for your undies in a wire bin, a hat box, or a velvet-lined drawer.

Statistics say women wear one-tenth of the clothes in their closet. I'd have to say that's on the high side.

Phase III: Tough Love

Cleaning out your closet will free your clothes to get more friendly with each other. When you take out what you don't love anymore, what isn't beautiful to you or what you've outgrown, then all that's left in there are possible playmates. Your brown skirt can look along the closet pole, spot your ivory ruffled blouse, and beg to go out together. Before the editing, they'd never have had a chance to meet. When you weed out the ordinary, the blah, and the unpleasant, you feel abundance with the clothes that remain. Now that's a friendly closet!

Having a closet full of *fresh, grand, and lovely choices* where each piece nourishes you takes clarity and firmness — two things that challenge women when it comes to clothes. We make all kinds of excuses for clothes like: "Oh, but it'll come back someday" or "but there's still some wear left in these twenty-year-old jeans" or "but my mother-in-law gave it to me, I can't throw it away."

It's time to practice "tough love." You must be brave. Dollar signs will jump in front of you like ghosts as you face unwise past purchases. You might hear yourself say, "What was I thinking?" It will be easy to get down on yourself. Stop. You didn't know better. Now you do. In the past, it was okay to buy something that was just okay. That's not true anymore. We're changing all that now.

Using a Buddy

Here's a preview of how this editing step works so you can plan whether to have your buddy along or to do it alone. You could break this up into a few steps you do on your own and then bring your buddy in as the closer. Remember, the closer is the fresh pitcher that the manager puts in near the end of the game to bring in the win. Your buddy can be a closer and help you get a winning wardrobe by throwing the third strike on the expired clothes in your closet.

When you are at this step, your buddy may say something like the following as she holds up each item:

Attention buddies: If your friend says, "But it hasn't worn out yet," remind her that her husband's god-awful orange tie-dye shirt from the 1970s hasn't worn out either!

"When was the last time you wore this?"

"How do you feel when you put this on?"

"Does this fit you now?"

"On a scale of 1 to 10, where does this item lie?"

"Is it the memory of this item that you're attached to, or the item itself?"

Gentle logic can sometimes dislodge a weak excuse for hanging onto something. When she insists, "But it might come back," agree with her. You could say, "Yes, it will come back — later in the century, when your body is different, when you've changed political parties, when little children are calling you Grandma — or Great Grandma."

The Clean-out in 10 Steps

Oh boy! Here we go! Ready? Crank up the volume on the CD. Only ten steps to a clean closet. Let's go!

STEP 1 **Everything that's not part of your current working wardrobe finds a new home.** Your closet is your personal shrine to getting dressed. That means everything that's not clothes gets removed. Art projects, sporting equipment, file boxes, etc. Remove them now!

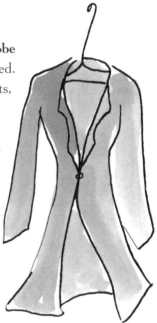

STEP 2 **All empty shopping bags, empty shoe boxes and plastic dry-cleaning bags get tossed.** So do the three dozen random empty hangers that have collected in there. We are creating space and breathing room. Can you see the floor yet?

STEP 3 **Work on one season, fall/winter or spring/summer, at a time.** Take out all the things that you'll wear six months from now. It's just too much to deal with your full wardrobe at one time unless you have obsessive-compulsive tendencies, which many of us have. In that case, go ahead and tackle the whole thing. But don't waste a lot of time on decisions about clothes from the season opposite the one you're in. You don't even know who you'll be next season, let alone whether those brown wool pants will still thrill you. Pull "other" season items out of your working closet and store them somewhere else — in another closet or in a box.

NOTE: When you edit your closet, it's great to pull things out completely. If you can get a portable clothes rack to set up in your room, do it. Pull a section out (blouses, skirts, pants, jackets) and work on a category at a time. Clothes look very different outside of the closet. We are less attached to them and can face them more honestly when they are in the light of day. Which reminds me — plan to do this early in the day when you have plenty of good light in the room where you're working. Dark rooms can impede your progress.

STEP 4 **Pull out clothes that are: expired, a bad color, ripped, stained or just don't fit.** Yes, take them out. Your closet contains expired clothes. It's time to remove them. They're out-of-date. If their counterparts were to make a comeback in a future decade, they'd appear in fabrics made from new technologies, so yours would still be out-of-date.

Feeling resistant? Okay, sit down. It's time we had a little chat. Think of it this way. If clothes were like dairy products and had expiration dates written along their side seams, wouldn't it be so much easier to throw them out once they had gone bad? Deep down, you know which clothes have expired! They are has-beens that once were the height of style. They used to hang there fresh and proud, but now just hang and droop. They aren't fit to adorn your body anymore, and if they were food, they'd surely have turned colors by now, shrunk two sizes, and smell very strange.

So you must go through your closet and separate the fresh, unspoiled clothes from those that have expired. This is not cruel! In order to see and use the clothes that are current and flattering, you have to be able to find them. Besides, wearing out-of-date clothes makes you look out-of-date and you're not.

You aren't wearing those clothes anyway, or if you are, are you enjoying them? Tell the truth. **Maybe it's time to let go.** They served you once, just like that couch of yours before the cat peed on it and it had to be taken to the dump. That floral print party dress with the big shoulder pads and the puffy sleeves had its time. Those stirrup pants had their glory. Life moves on, seasons change, so do you and the clothes in your closet.

At the same time, face the color truth. Pull out once and for all the clothes that clash with your coloring. You know which things you never reach for because your pale skin looks green when you wear it or it turns your auburn hair orange? These are the ones that have everyone wanting to take your temperature because that shade of yellow makes you look ill. Bad color choices bring you down. Put them in your give-away pile and let someone else benefit. Your closet should be full of colors that compliment what nature gave you.

Also, as you examine each item of clothing in your closet, tell the truth about stains. If you have a bleach stain on a sleeve or a spot that won't come out, toss these items now. They've expired.

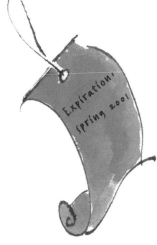

DO CLOTHES EXPIRE LIKE DAIRY PRODUCTS? YES! If they were food, they'd surely smell very strange.

Comb through your closet and pull out all the things that don't fit you. This closet is about serving the body you are currently in. If you are someone who consistently fluctuates in weight at that time of the month (we are women after all) allow your closet to accommodate a couple of body sizes. But beyond that, darn it, get those clothes out of there that don't fit you! No trophy clothes belong in your closet. I've seen those size 6 jeans that women keep to remind them of a size they once were. Let it go! **Get current!** Be in present time! I've also heard of women having smaller clothes in their closet for "incentive." To remind them of what they want to be fitting into . . . someday. Can you do that reminding somewhere else? What's in your closet now fits you now and serves you now. Is that clear?

If you have something precious in there AND you keep it because of sentiment, not size, then consider putting it in your souvenir box — that pretty box you bought to store the things that you'll never wear but you never want to forget.

These are headed for your clothing museum. They've moved beyond clothing; now they're conversation pieces. Either fold them gingerly and place them in that lovely box or hang them in one of those portable canvas hanging storage units. Put them in another closet, away from your working closet. Or be creative. Hang them up as art pieces where you can show them off and continue to enjoy them.

STEP 5 **Separate your discards and deal with ambivalent clothes.** As you weed through your closet, you'll come across things you just aren't sure of. Pull them out and come back to them at the end of the clean-out, or when your buddy shows up to help you. Start getting used to seeing only the things you love.

Some things may be obvious to you — what needs to be tossed, what needs to be altered — but sometimes it takes another set of eyes to get to the truth of a piece of clothing. Call up your buddy. She could be the tie-breaker with the courage to say, "Look my friend, you haven't worn that in years AND it's not really your color AND if you look at the sleeve, you'll see your elbow poking through where it's not supposed to!" God help you if you still manage to hang onto it. Remember, *it feels SO GOOD to let go.*

> **You won't have to go through this ever again because you are learning how to buy things that are just right for you!**

Here are some questions to ask as you face that ambivalent pile. Remember, **tell the truth!**

Do I love it?

Does it serve my current life?

Does it fit me now?

Does it bring me up or bring me down to wear it?

Start your own clothing museum for the clothes that really mean something to you sentimentally.

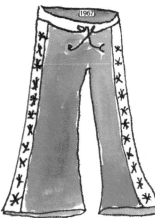

Look at your discards. Are some things in good enough shape that to go to a consignment store? Put those in a shopping bag with their destination attached to the bag. Do you have some things a friend or relative would like? Put them in a shopping bag with their name on it. Do you have some clean, wearable and in good condition clothes that you want to take to a charity? Good, calculate their value and put them in a bag with the name of their new home taped to it. And then there are things you just need to toss. You don't want them, your relatives don't want them, the consignment store doesn't want them. No one wants them. Put them out of their misery and put them in a trash bag.

STEP 6 **Pull out all the clothes that need mending.** Hems that have fallen, buttons that are hanging, seams that have opened. Maybe there's a blouse that once you've changed the buttons, you'll love. Make a mending pile. What needs altering? Maybe you've changed size and something needs to be taken in before you can wear it again. Make an alterations pile. When will you have finished these tasks? Put the date from your schedule on top of the pile and put it on your calendar as well. If you don't have a good alterations person, make a note and start asking your friends for referrals.

STEP 7 **Breathe.** Even though you are looking into your closet now and wondering where all your clothes went. Remember, the truth is you haven't been wearing those things you've pulled out — the not-me-any-mores, the bad-fit clothes, the clothes that needed mending. Nothing is wrong, everything is right. Take your courage pill and lean on me. I've been there. I've seen closets that had three hanging items once the rejects left. Don't forget, you ARE going to replace things. And you'll be so much smarter when you do.

STEP 8 **Sort through your drawers of clothes.** Most people have drawers that hold a multitude of sins — sock drawers, underwear drawers, workout drawers, scarf drawers, T-shirt drawers. I don't know why it is so hard to go through these drawers and get rid of socks that have no mates, or underwear that you'll only wear if your washing machine breaks down. Face these ills! I want you to feel nothing but good when you open those drawers.

Get the ratty panties into the garbage. Pair up those socks and discard the singles. Go through your hosiery drawer and get rid of all the colors you never wear. I know you have twelve pairs of unopened ivory hose. Get rid of them. Put them in your bag to go to charities if that makes you feel better.

Go through your handbags and tell the truth. Some are just trashed, some are out-of-date, some of them you just don't like. Get them out. Go through your exercise wear and face the fact that **you don't need thirty-four running T-shirts.** Pick out a favorite baker's dozen or less. There's no need to injure a shoulder trying to close the workout drawer in your dresser.

STEP 9 **Putting your closet back together.** Ahh, now doesn't that feel so much better? Take a break and peer into that lovely closet of yours. Wow! Get out the vacuum cleaner and vacuum the floor. Dust the shelves. Assess the lighting situation. Do you need a brighter bulb, a different fixture? Call a handyman or woman to help you get more light in there if your closet is dim. Hang bags of lavender or put orange peels on a shelf to give it a nice aroma. Sip something refreshing. *You're doing great!*

Now we're going to start putting things back together again. Don't start until you've caught your breath, had a bit of nourishment and slipped another CD into your player. If you're with your buddy, give each other some high fives. Ready? Okay, here we go.

All your hangers are going to be the same. It has a calming effect to open up your closet and see all the same hangers. It's like looking at a

Trash it! If you don't want them, your relatives don't want them, the consignment stores don't want them. NO ONE wants them.

lawn and seeing only green grass without brown spots or twelve varieties of weeds thrown in. You are *weeding out* the mismatched hangers and replacing them with matching ones either plastic coated metal hangers or plastic tubular hangers in your favorite color. Wire hangers from the dry cleaners are really bad for your clothes which need more support than they offer. Take them back to the dry cleaners. Rehang all your clothes on your new hangers and head everything in the same direction.

Organize the clothes in your closet by color, dark to light. Just as it's delightful to open up a box of crayons and see all the colors in order, it's *easy on the eyes* to see your clothes grouped that way. Organize by color and then arrange by item — coats, pants, blazers, long-sleeved blouses, short-sleeved tops. It's easy to see what your color habits are. If black takes up three-quarters of your closet, it may be time to consider adding color to your wardrobe.

Put as much as possible in plain sight. So many people forget what they have because they can't see it. Here's where you can have fun with storage containers. Take your storage units and neatly arrange your clothes and accessories in them. If you have a shelf above your closet pole, stack T-shirts, jeans, sweaters and so forth up there. A rectangular basket can sit on its side and store handbags. Hang a shoe rack over the back of a closet door. Hat boxes can hold scarves or underwear.

Use a storage box to hold your travel items. Anytime you're going on a trip, you can pull out the box with your leak-proof cosmetic bag, your shoe bags, mini-toiletries, umbrella, travel raincoat, etc., and you're ready to go.

REMINDERS: Put your style words, vision, or collages on the closet door or an inside shelf. Keep these reminders of what you're moving toward in a visible place to stay inspired while you develop new wardrobe muscles.

STEP 10 **Take an inventory.** If it's midnight and you've been at it for twelve hours and are exhausted, then it's time for bed. This next step should happen tomorrow or at your next scheduled closet date. If you are energized by your closet clean-out, then you could be flying high and may want to just jump right into this next step. Great either way. With all the clutter out of the way, you're ready to study what's left and build some outfits.

Go through all the categories of clothes. Get out pen and paper. How many pairs of pants do you own? Skirts? Dresses? Coats? Sweaters? Blouses? Tops? This is like checking the pantry before you go shopping. Do you have twelve jars of tomato sauce and no pasta? Before you buy any more pants, see if you've got the tops to go with the ones you already own. By counting you know exactly where your wardrobe's strengths and weaknesses are. Are you strong in shoes and weak in coats? Great with pants, awful with tops? Often people have things that are easy for them to shop for, but then other areas of their wardrobe suffer. Maybe you focus on sweaters because that way you can avoid the challenge of finding a good fit in pants. What's suffering in your wardrobe?

Make some notes. What needs your immediate attention?

FOCUS
What's suffering in your wardrobe? Often people have things that are easy for them to shop for, but then other areas of their wardrobe suffer.

FILL IN THE BLANKS:

I have plenty of _____

_____

I'm missing _____

_____

The areas that need to be handled first are

_____

_____

_____

_____

What are the staples in your wardrobe? Often there are a handful of items that are the glue that holds everything else together in your wardrobe. What are those things that if they disappeared tomorrow would leave you stranded in your house with nothing to wear? My staples are a jean jacket, a stretchy boot, a black camisole, two pairs of pants in black and brown and a tote bag that fits my files perfectly. Recognize your staples now and **get them on a shopping list.** You need to replace these babies or back them up for wardrobe security. It's like backing up files on your computer. If that hard drive goes, you're in trouble.

MY STAPLES ARE:

_____

_____

_____

_____

Just a reminder

Review your clothes giveaway day. Is this date reasonable? If not, make a new plan and follow through. Don't forget your alterations and repair day. You'll feel like you have a new wardrobe once your alterations come home.

TRY THIS:

Have a swap meet in your living room. In an effort to find homes for your discards, invite your friends over and have them bring theirs as well. Toss everything on the living room floor, or if you want to be more civilized, set up a portable rack and let the trading begin. But remember, the same standards hold as before. You have to love it before it goes home with you. Whatever remains goes to your favorite charity. One client of mine also invited her friends to bring all their leftover face, hair, and body products that hadn't been used and swap those as well.

The Finale — Celebrating and Photos

Okay, now's the time you've been waiting for: the celebration! I'm so proud of you! Get out your camera. Photograph your closet for the "after" pictures. Celebrate with your buddy. Sit at your beautiful shrine. Propose a toast. Great job! You might even want to rent a movie and share some popcorn with your buddy. Pick a movie with some good closet scenes.

CONGRATS!

Putting Your Look Together

YOUR CLOSET IS AS ORGANIZED now as a professional chef's kitchen. Just as the chef's pots and pans hang all shiny and within reach, so do your belts, handbags, and scarves. The way the spices are organized alphabetically, your clothes are sorted according to color. Just as the chef knows what's in her pantry, you know what's in your closet because you took an inventory. A chef gathers her recipes, decides what she's going to cook, prepares her menu, and then shops for the ingredients she's missing.

I'm not a professional chef, but I do eat every day. The most efficient I've ever been in the kitchen was when I sat down with my kids and we planned our meals for the week. We checked the pantry to see what we had, made a shopping list of what we needed, shopped, and then prepared the meals accordingly. We were never happier.

When you work your wardrobe with that same kind of efficiency, you'll be happy too. Getting dressed is so effortless when you follow the steps I've outlined in this chapter.

By spending several hours in your closet putting outfits together and recording them either in writing or in pictures, we're going to plan your wardrobe for a season. By taking a day to do this, you'll have outfits to choose from all season long. **Think of it — a day of planning equals a season of wearing!** We'll find out exactly what you need to add to your wardrobe to consistently make outfits that fit your style recipe. If an outfit has most of the ingredients but is missing something, that "something" will go on your shopping list. After we've made lots of outfits, you'll have a concise shopping list to take with you to the stores. When you find those items you'll be able to complete all the outfits that you come up with today. It's easy!

Okay, you've got your style recipe and the pictures you pulled from magazines and catalogs to guide you. You're ready to get into your closet to mix and blend your ingredients and cook up a fabulous wardrobe for the season that will nourish and satisfy you.

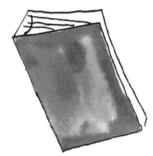

YOU'LL NEED:
1. **20–30 copies of Brenda's Wardrobe Workout Chart (see pg. 128)**
2. **Your style recipe (see pg. 74)**
3. **Your collages**
4. **Blank paper**
5. **Your binder**
6. **Sheet protectors**

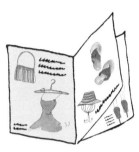

HAVE ON HAND:
1. **A full-length mirror**
2. **A portable clothes rack (if you have one)**
3. **Refreshments**
4. **Your buddy (if you're using one)**

BUDDY EXERCISES:

Here's what your buddy can do for you on your building outfits day:

1. Your buddy can help you stay on track. She helps keep some sense of order in the room so you don't bury prized possessions and not find them until next Tuesday.

2. Your buddy can review your style words and ask you if the way you feel in the outfits matches your words. Your buddy's questions, comments, and clarifications help you stay true to your style recipe and resist old patterns.

3. Your buddy can offer suggestions: Try this jacket on. How about these flat shoes instead of the heels? Maybe the red sweater would be better.

4. Your buddy can reinforce your good work: "Wow! That looks so great on you!"

5. Your buddy can point out what's missing. "You need a brown belt for this." She writes "brown belt" on your shopping list along with the outfit it will be purchased for. Buddies make it easier.

BRENDA'S WARDROBE WORKOUT CHART

KEY PIECE

SEASON:_____

	1	2	3	4	5
Top					
Outerwear (Jacket, Sweater, Coat)					
Footwear (Shoes, Socks, Hose)					
Underwear					
Accessories (Handbag, Belt, Scarf, Jewelry)					

Working the Chart

As you put outfits together, you'll be writing down every part of each outfit on Brenda's Wardrobe Workout Chart. I've been using these with my clients for years. One chart documents up to five complete outfits. On the opposite page is a sample Wardrobe Workout Chart. Before you write in the one provided, make copies. Pretty soon, you'll have a binder full of these!

Let me show you how it works. On the top right fill in the season you're working in — spring, summer, winter, fall, or transition (that time between summer and fall or winter and spring when the weather is more unpredictable). I like to write in the date that we create these outfits. Just the month and the year is adequate. You can note the date right under the line for "season." It's another reference as you build your wardrobe from year-to-year.

In the large box at the top left write the key piece around which you'll **build outfits.** This is a bottom piece from your wardrobe — a specific pair of pants, skirt, shorts — or a dress. If you have three pairs of black pants, give each pair distinction. You can distinguish it by fabric content (cotton, linen, wool, silk), function (dressy, casual, play, work), designer, or the store you bought it from.

There are five columns to accommodate five different outfits. On the left margin you'll see a box for every part of the outfit — top, outerwear, footwear, underwear, accessories. Once completed, you'll have up to five outfits using that same bottom. If you're working with a dress, put the dress in the box and fill in the whole Wardrobe Workout Chart except for the row for "top."

As you **create** an outfit, you might want to note at the top of each column the occasion you'll be wearing it. For instance, two columns of outfits made with your lightweight wool black pants may be for work and three columns for dates. Otherwise, you can create one Wardrobe Workout Chart just for work that uses the lightweight wool black pant as the key piece and one chart with "date" outfits made from the same pant if it's that versatile. You can note "date" or "work" under "Season."

Once you've worked through the "bottoms" in your wardrobe and the charts are filled in, slip them into plastic sheet protectors and put them in your binder. You can also separate your Wardrobe Workout Charts by occasion. Use your dividers and make categories

Don't write on your Wardrobe Workout Chart —yet! Make copies first. Pretty soon, you'll have a binder full of these!

that work for you. You can divide your charts by activity — work clothes, play clothes, social/event clothes, weekend clothes, or divide by season — fall, winter, spring, summer, transition. You'll refer to these charts all season long and then make new ones next season.

Your binder full of outfits will be a lifesaver!

If you've written an outfit down, you know it exists. All of us wake up some mornings and our brains can't figure out what to wear. That's when it's great to flip through your binder and effortlessly find something to wear.

A SPECIAL TIP: If you are more of a visual person and need to see it in pictures, document your outfits on film. Lay the clothes out with the shoes and other accessories on the bed and photograph them. If you are missing important ingredients for an outfit, it's best to wait until after your shopping trip to photograph it. Whatever you do, don't put yourself in the photo. If the snapshot is less than favorable you could focus on a bad photo and not the outfit. Come on! Snapshots are most often NOT flattering. I don't want you ignoring the cool outfit because you got distracted by your hair, hips, legs, or arms.

Creating Outfits

Make categories that work for YOU. Divide clothes by activity or seasons.

Okay, let's start cooking! Set up your portable clothes rack or use an ironing board as a rack. Put your full-length mirror in a well-lit spot. I'm saying it again: You MUST have a full-length mirror. You need to view yourself from head to toe, front to back, taking in the wonderful work of art you're creating. Standing on a chair or crouching in front of a bathroom mirror is not acceptable. Since we are making complete outfits, pull out your accessories — scarves, belts, shoes, hats, earrings, bracelets, necklaces — and have them in full view.

Grab a Wardrobe Workout Chart. Pull a pant or skirt from your closet. Let's do a practice one with a wool plum colored trouser. Give it a specific name and write it in the "key piece" box.

KEY PIECE
wool plum trousers

Go through your closet and pull out all the tops that could conceivably be worn with those plum trousers. Put them all on your rack, or throw them in a stack on your bed. Slip into the plum trouser and, one-by-one, start trying on tops. What looks great to you? Is there something about the combination of pant and top that fits your style recipe? If your recipe calls for "lively," then seek out a top that will make a lively statement, like maybe an orange shiny blouse. If your recipe calls for "sophistication," then you might want a matching plum blouse. Don't be quick to reject any possible tops until you've tried them on. Be open to surprises!

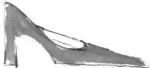

Once you've settled on a top that works, figure out what jacket, coat or sweater goes with it. A different outer piece can definitely change the look of the outfit. There's a **big difference** between a motocross leather jacket and a sequined cardigan sweater. The whole outfit may be the same except for the outer piece. Honor each outfit with its own column even if that means changing only one thing. As you see, you could have lots of distinctively different combinations with only slight variations in content.

Try on several pairs of shoes with the outfit. When you've got it, stop and write it all down.

Try on several pairs of shoes with the outfit. Note what socks or hosiery you'll wear. Look at your accessories. How are you going to finish this outfit? **Accessories really distinguish an outfit.** So what earrings, necklaces, bracelets are you going to wear? Will you add a scarf? What handbag will you wear? You may have tried on several different combinations before you've pulled it all together and the bells are ringing. When they do, stop and write it all down.

Don't forget the undies. Some pants need thong underwear to work or they don't work at all! Some skirts need "smoothies," those undergarments that have built-in panels that smooth out body parts. Some knit tops need smooth cup bras so the knit looks smooth and not bumpy (from patterned lace bras). Make those notes now so you won't forget when it comes time to wear that outfit.

You may put an outfit together that works, but doesn't have the energy of your style words. So scratch that one. Record only those outfits you love to see on yourself and just can't wait to wear. These are the outfits that reflect **the most current version of yourself** and are flattering to you.

Work with all the possible tops that could go with that pant before you move onto the next bottom. By the time you're done working with that plum pant, you may have twelve outfits that go with it — surely many more than you ever imagined. That's the way it goes.

The reason you write everything down is so you won't forget. You probably knew that. But people just as smart as you start out creating outfits they love and they think they'll remember each one because the outfits are so great. They are great. Each one will probably be your new favorite. That's why it's just too hard to remember them all. I've spent four hours at a time in clients' closets and at the end of our session, when they needed to go to work, they were completely baffled by what to wear. At the same time they're having a blast seeing all these new outfits coming together, it's mentally exhausting. So please, oh please, don't think you're that smarty pants who will remember everything. There will be dozens of great outfits, so write them down. You can thank me later.

As you put outfits together, there are things that will be missing. Write "shopping list" on a blank sheet of paper. An outfit you're working on may need a cute sandal in red to really set it off. Put that red sandal on your shopping list. As you build the outfit, you can record the "red sandal" in the footwear box in pencil as if it were complete. Or put an asterisk on that item you need to shop for.

As a shopping list develops, keep your notes detailed. Note the item you're shopping for and what it's supposed to go with. Believe me, if you don't, it's so easy to forget your great idea. You're taking an in-depth look at your wardrobe for the first time ever. There's so much to keep track of. I've seen it happen. Three days later you look at your shopping list and one of the items is "gold scarf." "Okay," you say, "I was going to get a gold scarf . . . but for what? I forget!" More notes than fewer is best.

As you're creating outfits, keep a close eye on the condition of your clothes. You may need to alter a pair of pants — take the waist in if you've lost some weight or let the waist out if you've gained some weight. WARNING: If this pushes a button for you, remember it's time to focus on clothes and how they fit, not on your weight. Remember "Fit First"! Write "To Do" at the top of another sheet of paper. Keep your to do list handy. You may want to upgrade the buttons on a shirt, shorten a skirt, taper the legs on pants. Write down what needs what and set a date to take care of your alterations, preferably, within the week.

Keep building outfits! The more efficient you are at this stage of your wardrobe planning, the smarter you'll be in the shopping stage. You should be solving some mysteries, like why you never wear that tweed pant — because you really need an olive shoe to go with it! Or why a certain accessory is about to fall apart — because it goes with everything in your wardrobe (and should immediately go on your shopping list so you have a replacement).

Don't forget to accentuate the positive. As you're creating outfits, stand in front of your mirror. Are you bringing focus to the parts of your face and body that you wanted to? Your buddy can help you with this.

Irresistibly your style words are flying out of your or your buddy's mouth. As you create outfits, you'll both be exclaiming, "Oh my gosh! That is so (fill in the blank with the appropriate style word, such as sophisticated! playful! dramatic! sexy!)."

8 Tips for Creating Great Looks

Pay attention to these tips so you get a great put together look that keeps the focus on your assets. Study yourself in the mirror, or ask you buddy to give you feedback.

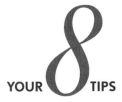

YOUR 8 TIPS

1. Focus on the face
2. Follow the eye
3. Copy scale
4. Consider hair
5. Duplicate pattern
6. Repeat coloring
7. Create themes
8. Combine fabrics

1. **Bring the focus to the face.** Always look for ways to do this — with a scarf, a necklace with a stone the same color as your eyes, great earrings, a fur collar, a jacket that pulls out highlight colors in your hair.

2. **Always follow how the eye travels up your body.** If you put together bright red pants and a black sweater, work that red back up to your face (unless your hair is the same shade of red), which will move the eye up your body. You can wear red lipstick or hang a red pendant around your neck. Or wear a print scarf that has red in it. If you wear a print on your bottom half, pick a color from the print and bring it up — again, in a lipstick, eye shadow, a necklace, earrings, eyeglass frames, scarf, or a pin. **Try this.** See if you have shoes, a belt (if you wear belts) and a handbag that match the general tones of your hair

because that will keep the eye moving up your body. For instance, if you have brown hair, you can wear a black long skirt and black T-shirt with brown sandals and a brown belt. The browns lead the eye straight up the body. This will blow your mind! It looks so cool.

3. **Look at your self and make "scale" connections.** Match the size (scale) of your features to the size (scale) of your clothes or accessories. If you have large features, look for accessories with large details — large-scale earrings or a bag or a belt with a large buckle on it. If you have delicate features, pull out a delicate necklace from your jewelry box or choose a blouse from your closet with delicate detailing like tiny rows of tucks. By repeating your "scale," you look even more like yourself!

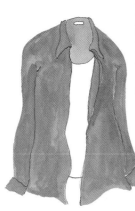

4. **Match the weight of your hair.** A person with thin, wispy hair wears lightweight or sheer fabrics easily, in layers for warmth. Someone with thick, coarse hair looks great in fabrics that have more weight to them — heavier cotton knits, wool or corduroy.

See how "right" you look when the fabrics you wear relate to the weight of your hair.

5. **Repeat the pattern of your skin and hair in fabrics.** If your hair and skin are smooth, you'll look great in smooth fabrics. If you have a lot of texture in your hair or skin, you'll look great in clothes that have texture. Match the texture of your skin and hair to the texture in your clothes.

6. **Repeat your coloring (hair, skin, or eyes) in your clothes.** If you are completely missing clothes in your coloring, think of some colors to put on your shopping list. Dark brown to black-haired women wear black easily. Ash-haired women look great in rosy taupes. Honey blonds look great in camel. Gray-haired women look great in shades of gray. Consider wearing shoes and belts that repeat your hair color. Then look at eye color! Repeating eye color is great for good communication. Colors that are close to eye colors draw us in and keep our attention.

7. **Cluster accessories to match a theme.** To help you out, think of the movies. If you watch a movie like Jane Austen's *Pride and Prejudice,* you don't expect Martians or robots to appear in an upcoming scene. All things in an authentic romantic period movie **relate to one another.** The robots and Martians would have their own movie theme, like sci-fi.

It's the same with accessories. Wild and zany (colorful polka dot socks, a big red wristwatch with live-looking hands, a lively striped handbag) is a theme that doesn't mix with classic (gold watch, gold fine-chain choker, gold knot earrings). Also remember that there needs to be one main focal point and all the other accessories play supporting roles, just like in the movies. Let a colorful pendant necklace be the main star. Wear earrings that pick up a color in the necklace but don't compete for center stage. Make sure the accessories have a similar feel or repeat a texture. That makes them good as supporting roles.

8. **When mixing fabrics, combine similar weights.** Thick corduroy pants are great with a chunky cable-knit turtleneck and heavy oxfords. A sheer top and jacket work well with a double layered fluid chiffon skirt and strappy sandals. Or if you are more creative or eclectic, you can use "disharmony" to express your style. Or you might enjoy combining dissimilar weights, like a lace blouse with a corduroy pant or a heavy boot with a chiffon skirt.

Remember that there needs to be one main focal point and all the other accessories play supporting roles.

BUDDY EXERCISE:

Make a date with your buddy (or your buddy team if you have one) to gather in front of the TV for the next major awards show — the Emmy's, Grammy's, Oscars, Golden Globes, etc. Study the actresses and look for the ones that get it right. For instance, look at how an actress will play up her coloring by matching her gown to her hair color. Anyone remember how Goldie Hawn did it by wearing a light gold sequined gown that pointed right to her golden blond head? Remember the year that Joan Allen wore a blue gown that made her eyes look as blue as the sky? Look at how an actress wears a gown that repeats the shape of a facial feature. One year Minnie Driver wore a gown whose neckline mimicked her jawline. It looked terrific! As each actress walks up to accept her award, study to see if she's repeating something about her coloring, scale, texture or an aspect of her personality. Come up with style words that you think match the stars. It sharpens your own understanding of the style words you and your friends use for yourselves.

Ever think of mixing pond scum, wheat fields, and tall weeds in your wardrobe? Take a field trip and see how nature puts colors together.

TRY THIS:

Notice how nature blends colors together. I suggest you get out of the city limits and into the countryside. Look at tree bark and leaves. Get inspired by a sunrise or a sunset or the colors in a rainstorm. Bring a note pad with you and go hunting for color combos that you can take home and try with clothes in your wardrobe. Here are a few combinations I discovered on a drive through Minnesota in October.

ivory (country churches)
black (tilled earth)
camel (faded cornfields) or caramel (wheat fields)

moss green (pond scum)
harvest gold (wheat fields)
rust (tall weeds near Star Lake)

cranberry (sumac)
eggplant (sunset colors in the sky)
tobacco brown (spent sunflower fields)

tobacco brown (ditch weeds)
honey (other ditch weeds)
green (grass)

red brown (end-of-the season sunflower fields)
honey (wheat fields)
pistachio green (that pond scum again)

black (plowed earth)
cranberry (sumac)
ivory (the prairie churches)

How are you doing? If you aren't hearing gleeful sounds coming from your closet, let's see what's going on. You may not have the right things to work with. That's okay. At least by trying to create outfits, you'll see what's missing. Some people have very short shopping lists and some people have long ones. Just keep telling the truth.

Study the pictures you pulled back in Get the Picture. If you don't feel like your look is coming together, the pictures might give you a clue as to why. Maybe you have the crisp white blouse in your closet, but your jeans are seven years old and don't have that sharp look only a new pair of jeans (like the ones in your picture) can give. Jeans rarely wear out but always need updating. It can make all the difference.

Often people have lots of clothes but don't have many accessories. Accessories often provide the personality that defines a look. Refer back to the Style Glossary and look up your style words. What accessories could you add to your shopping list that will really define your look? Think this through now so you won't get confused in the stores. If you have a good idea of what you're looking for, you have a great chance of finding it.

Flush Out Your Shopping List

You put your look together from the clothes in your closet or got as close as you could with what was there to work with. What's missing went on your shopping list. **Do you have areas that are a big void** — like you're taking yoga and you have no clothes to wear to class? Add "yoga outfit" to your list. Do you have nothing to wear when you're at home and just want to relax? Write "at home outfits" on your list. You don't necessarily need to know what those outfits will look like because you haven't been shopping for them in a long time, or ever! This may be the first time you actually take care of yourself in this category. That's okay. You can decide once you're at the store and you've looked around just what works best for you.

If you have a category that's pretty empty — let's use date clothes as an example — there are several levels to that category — casual dates, dressy dates, formal dates. Think through what you'd be happy to start with. Break it down as best you can. Maybe it would look like this:

THINGS NEEDING AN UPDATE QUICK:
1. Jeans
2. Shoes
3. Handbags
4. Haircuts
5. Hair color
6. Makeup

My Shopping List:

2 casual date outfits
(maybe great-fitting jeans
and a couple of sexy tops)

1 dressy date outfit
(a dress or dressy skirt)

Accessories that complete the outfits

A wrap for the evenings

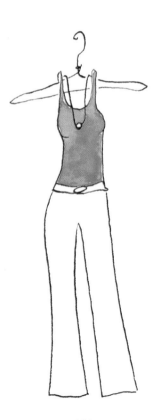

Now your shopping list has all the things you need to complete outfits and fill the gaps in your closet. You might not shop for everything at once, you may need to prioritize, but initially get everything on one list. However, you must also leave a slot on your list for the totally unexpected, for the something you'll fall in love with and just have to have. Add space for surprise and delight. It's not something you thought about. *It's a surprise!* You'll now it when you see it and you won't leave the store without it.

Maybe you'll come across an accessory that just delights you. Great! Fill that "delight" slot with something that makes you smile.

Can you see how all your work in Attitude Rehab and Get the Picture paid off here in your closet when you put your look together? The style recipe you created from your collages, exercises and interview gave you the road map so you can put things together in the way that supports how you're expressing yourself now. By editing the things from your closet that don't line up with your vision, it's easy to see what you already have that works, and what's missing from your wardrobe is clearly evident. Your shopping list is real rather than vague. Because you've spent time *really thinking* about your needs and wants, looking at your lifestyle to see what you actually need clothes for, and then taking an inventory of what's in your closet and what's not, you know where you're at! You can trust yourself to go shopping and fill your needs. Well, almost trust yourself. If you have any doubts about shopping, the tips in the next chapter will turn you into a pro.

Let's get ready to SHOP!

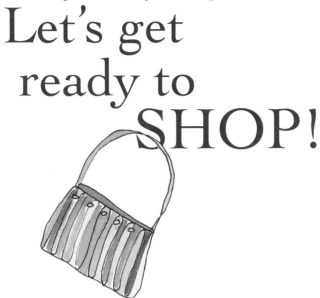

Shopping Fitness

PERSONAL TRAINERS EMPHASIZE HOW important it is to pace yourself when starting a new exercise program. It's the same with shopping. If you haven't been shopping for awhile and your shopping muscles are less than toned, you could overextend, or get burned out and frustrated without the proper training. Start out with some warm-up exercises. Here are some recommendations from a professional shopping coach, yours truly.

Warm-Up Exercises

Protect yourself. You know how when you go roller blading, you need to wear your knee pads and a helmet to protect yourself? Your fashion strategies will provide you with that kind of protection when you go shopping. There's nothing like standing in your bra and undies in a dressing room, under the glare of a cold fluorescent light, and looking at yourself in a carnival-quality mirror that distorts your thighs, to send you perilously close to a relapse, face first. Review the fashion strategies in Attitude Rehab until you can repeat after me with conviction: I'm not comparing. I'm worth full price. I focus on what works. I'm doing the love thing. I think "fit" first.

Work up to it. You don't go down the steepest hill first. You practice in your driveway. Call up your buddy, leave your cash at home and go for a trial run. Consider this your dress rehearsal. Take a spin through the stores and do some detective work. Walk through every department and get the lay of the land. Look for a salesperson who is working with someone in such a way that you get good vibes. Find out who she is and what days she works.

Train your eye to see what's ahead on the fashion track. The sooner you get acquainted with what's on the racks, the quicker your eye can get used to the latest looks and trends. The sooner you get on board with current looks, the longer you ride the fashion wave. So think of this as a research-and-development field trip before you take the one for real.

Shape your budget. You may have a budget of $250 or $10,000. Have an idea of what you're planning to spend. Make priorities. If your budget is limited, go to the biggest need first and fill it. If you've neglected shopping for a long time, start thinking about "sticker shock" before you face it head on. Prices have gone up and you could be very surprised.

Not only are you worth full price, you're worth taking all the time you need for shopping. You're only going to buy what you love and it may take a shopping trip or two to do that.

Whatever you budget, consider what would happen if you got out there and found more things you love than you'd ever imagine. On Cara's lucky shopping day we found four great **"must-have"** coats. One was a black slicker with a cute black-and-white striped lining, good for the rainy season. One was a divine quilted jacket in a chalk color, great for her sporty look. One was a long dressy cashmere coat with a hood perfect for going to the opera, ballet, or any special occasion. And the last one was a classic basic coat to wear to work.

All of her coats had died at the same time so she had use for every single one of these. We shopped in January taking advantage of great sale prices, but still, she hadn't anticipated finding four great coats at once.

Consider what would happen if that bumper crop was waiting for you out there. You'll be less anxious about spending more if you've already decided to cover the expense. And remember, if you haven't shopped in a long time and have some catching up to do you might want to be more generous with your budget.

Decide if shopping is a sport you prefer to do alone or with a buddy. A buddy in the dressing room will help you stay focused. She will hang up clothes and hunt for different sizes, provide you with sustenance when you need it, and will give you the power talk when you're on the last lap. She'll cheer you on and help make the day fun. Call on a buddy and pick a date and meeting place.

Take instruction from loving voices. Tune into my voice in your head. You'll hear me saying things like, "Remember, you're worth full price" and "Do you love it?" Or, "Dress for the body you are currently in."

THE NIGHT BEFORE: ROUNDING UP YOUR POSSE

O.K., here's what you want to gather together the night before you shop:

1. Your shopping list

2. Your key style words

3. A water bottle

4. Power bars

5. A notebook

6. Any items that need matching or mates to complete an outfit

7. Voices in your head (the good ones)

Then you'll have Bridget's voice. You'll want to listen to your alter ego character, because she'll help you *take risks.* You may also have your fashion heroine's voice steering you clear of ruts and bad habits to help you go for your new, improved look.

Don't shop without the loving voices in your head. Give any "bad" voices the day off. Make them stay home. Leave them some old videos, some popcorn, and set them on the couch in their faded worn sweats to watch TV all afternoon.

Don't shop without the loving voices in your head. Give any "bad" voices the day off!

Reminders from Your Shopping Coach

Every shopping athlete needs a shopping coach and I'm here for you! Shopping is quite a workout. I want you to be in tip-top shape so review these strategies before you embark on your big day. In fact, you might want to take these tips along with you so you can refer to them a few times throughout the day. Pack these proven power tips along with your power snacks and you're sure to have the most successful shopping trip you've ever had!

Save receipts. Slip them in a plastic zipper compartment with three side punches and store them in your binder. This gives you easy access as you decide what you're keeping and what you're returning. Knowing what you spend on your clothes will help you budget for them next year. You will have your receipts at a later date if something goes wrong with a garment and it needs to go back to the manufacturer.

Know the return policies of the stores where you shop. Department stores and big chains generally offer the most generous return policies. Be sure you know ahead of time what the policy is. If you shop in the bigger stores, they will usually stand firmly behind the products they offer. If you bought something that didn't hold up the way you expected or you followed the care instructions and got bad results, you can return it. The store sends it back to the manufacturer. Smaller boutiques have more limited return and exchange policies. The most restricted ones I've come across are five days/exchange only. This is tough at the beginning of your new process when you might not be confident about your decision-making. I like my clients to know they can take everything back tomorrow if they get freaked out.

Remember the cost-per-wear formula. Buying something for $100 that you wear one hundred times, costs you $1 per wearing. If you buy something for $100 and you wear it once, it cost you $100 per wear. It's much smarter to buy the more expensive thing that you wear to death than to buy the substitute for less that misses the mark and sits in your closet. Admit it, the dress that's thirty bucks more is the one you adore. In the past, you might have thought that the cheaper one was the smarter buy. Not anymore. Go for what you love. If that means paying more for it, then do it. It's worth it in the end.

If you have a lot of shopping needs, don't expect to satisfy them all in one day. Focus on one area — weekend play clothes, work clothes, special occasion dressing — at a time.

Know your shopping capacity. Schedule your shopping for a few evenings or a few mornings if you are working on your wardrobe for an entire season.

Practice my Three-Solutions-to-Any Problem Rule. If when shopping you get stuck thinking that there's ONE and only one thing that will make an outfit work, you limit yourself too much. Sometimes we see something in a magazine and decide only that exact item will do. It's great to go with an idea of what shoe you want to wear with your garden dress to your friend's party, but instead of insisting on that ONE solution, shop with the idea that three solutions are available. Be open and let more possibilities exist.

Fill in your wardrobe gaps first. When you fill the gaps, your wardrobe will expand like those tiny sponge lizards that when you put them in water grow thirty times their original size.

Buy clothes in colors that flatter you the minute you slip into them. It's the wise woman who has a closet full of clothes that make her look her best even when she isn't feeling that way.

Accessories: don't leave the store without them. They are the glue, the magic, the provocative pieces that individualize your style and set you apart from all the rest.

Buy trendy items in small doses. A scarf or a handbag in an animal print rather than a whole pant suit is a smaller investment in a trend that could be over in six months.

Remember, from now on, your relationship with clothes is like a marriage. Love and commit to them and they will bring you joy and pleasure.

Shopping Workout

Okay kids, fasten your seatbelts, we're going shopping. Let's double-check to be sure you're ready. You have your style recipe and

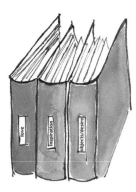

WRITE IT DOWN:
The worst place to keep a good thought is in your head!

your shopping list. You know what features and body parts you want to spotlight. You're ready to go!

STEP 1 **Leave the house looking your best.** Put some makeup on and style your hair. Wear good underwear, clothes, and shoes that are easy to get in and out of. Everything looks better and you feel better when you start the day looking good.

STEP 2 **Peruse and choose.** When you get to the store, check it out from department to department. Spend the first forty-five minutes or so looking through the racks pulling all likely candidates. If there are limits to what you can take into a dressing room, store the remainders on the racks provided near the dressing rooms. A smile is often all you need to get the cooperation of the person supervising the clothes.

STEP 3 **Keep order in the dressing room.** Take off your clothes and hang them up so they don't get crushed and buried. You want to walk out looking like you did when you came in.

STEP 4 **Try things on.** Make a reject pile, a maybe pile and a YES pile.

STEP 5 **Keep cleaning out the dressing room.** Get the rejects back on the hangers and return them to the salesperson who is helping you, or turn this step over to your buddy.

STEP 6 **Ask good questions.** Do this with the YES clothes first, and then carefully go over the items about which you aren't 100 percent sure. Reason things out with clarifying questions:

Do you like the fit but not the color?

Do you like the color but the fabric is too high maintenance for you?

Would it be better in another size?

Is the color flattering?

Does it hang right or does it twist on your body?

Does this make you feel great or just so-so?

Does this item fit your style words?

Do you look in the mirror and see your "Bridget"?

Are you looking at a clearer vision of yourself?

Do these items fit the bill for what you were looking for?

Do you love it?

Under pressure you're more likely to buy "what'll do". Limited time limits your shopping choices.

And finally, do you want to marry it? Do you remember how as little kids we said this to each other on the playground? We'd say, "Well, if you love it, then marry it." Play with me for a minute. Do you want to marry this item? I'm using that playground line to measure your commitment to this piece of clothing. Just as it's easier to get married than unmarried, it's a lot easier to add things to a wardrobe and a lot harder to get rid of them. You saw that when we did your closet. So think about that now. **Are you ready to commit** to caring for this item as long as it shall last? There's that sweater. You know you'd do anything for that sweater, including mending, dry cleaning, and storing it properly. But some sweaters you put on, you take off, and throw in a heap with little respect at all. Remember, from now on, your relationship to clothes is like a marriage. Love and commit to them and they will bring you joy and pleasure.

STEP 7 **Take time outs.** Are you getting tired? Need a break? Keep drinking water. Get something to eat if you need to. Ask your salesperson to hang onto your things while you step out for some fresh air. Make a trip to the ladies room.

ROME WASN'T BUILT IN A DAY If you have a lot of shopping needs, don't expect to solve them overnight. Focus on one area at a time.

STEP 8 **Put things on hold.** Some people like to go from store to store and hunt and gather. If this is your style, have your items put on hold. It's a good idea to hold your items longer than you think you'll need to . . . just in case. You may make your decisions at the end of the day, or you may want to go home and sleep on it. You may want to bring your buddy back the next day for a second opinion.

STEP 9 **Take notes while you're in the dressing room.** You may buy an outfit in separates that you adored in the dressing room but once you're home, you forgot how it all went together. Remember what you adored and write it down. You can get mentally exhausted if you spend hours in a dressing room.

Keep pages in your journal for **To Do Soon, To Buy Later,** or **To Try at Home.** Capture all those thoughts while you're having them. As my friends, Sunny and Gary Yates always say, the worst place to keep a good idea is in your head.

Have you discovered a really cute outfit AND it needs black sandals to complete it? Take out that notebook and **write this down.** Think about accessories, stockings, socks, shoes, handbags, hair ornaments, coats, jackets, shawls. If you don't have time to shop for the accessories on the same day, make notes for your next trip. Be sure to write down the item so it doesn't get lost in all the flurry and fun of shopping. Maybe your arms or legs need a tanning product to complete the sleeveless/bare legs outfit in order to look great. **Write that down.** Use your wardrobe journal to write down the questions that need answers once you're back home.

STEP 10 **Pay attention to what needs altering.** If you can, call in an alterations person from the store. If a pair of cotton pants requires laundering before hemming, then jot a note to yourself to bring the pants back after you've put them through the wash. If you fall in love with a top but hate the buttons, make a note to change them.

STEP 11 **Pace yourself, don't race.** If you've had enough for the day, pack it up. Leave the dressing room neat and tidy. Just because. Make notes in your journal about what's next to do. When you get home, take a look at your calendar and schedule times to finish. Now you have a sense about your energy level for this project and can schedule your time accordingly. You may be someone who pushes right through, or you may find it more manageable to break it into smaller pieces. Your way is the right way.

STEP 12 **Make your final decisions at home.** I like to take clients shopping where the return policy is generous. That way you don't have to make final decisions until you have the clothes at home where you can look at them under your own lighting, in front of your own mirror, for as long as you like. So on your shopping day, take all the strong contenders home. Don't narrow your choices for final decisions if you aren't sure. Put your purchase on a credit card and tell the salesperson you're taking these home to make final decisions. It's too hard for most of us to shop and make all the decisions on the same day.

Don't forget the accessories! They are the glue, the magic that sets you apart from all the rest.

See how you're feeling once you get home. If you feel you overextended yourself on your shopping trip, then go home. Hang up your items and leave them in your closet until you have the energy and enthusiasm to look at them. It's so easy to get tired from shopping and then pull things out of their bags the minute you get home, look at your purchases and wonder, "What was I thinking?" Let's sidestep that. Get some rest if you need to so when you look at your things it's with fresh eyes. OR, if you're still excited, you might want to do a fashion show for the gang at home.

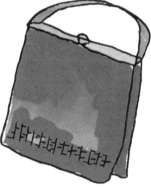

BUDDY EXERCISE:
Here are a few things you can ask your buddy to do for you on your shopping day.
1. Your buddy can help you face any excuses, rationalizations, internal saboteurs or stall tactics that could get in the way of getting the wardrobe you want and deserve.

2. If you say, "Oh well, at least it makes an outfit," your buddy can remind you that you are worth buying only what you love.

3. If you light up and then sink when you read the price tag, your buddy can remind you of the cost-per-wear formula. If you love it, you will wear it a lot.

4. Your buddy can help you with decisions and ask clarifying questions.

5. After a day of shopping, celebrate with your buddy! You can tell her how you feel. And if you're overwhelmed, she can remind you that you can always take everything back. You can talk about the highs and lows. Dream together about what pieces will go with what you have.

JUST FOR FUN:

Play fashion show. When my mother went shopping with me, we would always have a fashion show once the packages were brought into the house. "Go show your dad," she would say. She was always as happy for me as I was! There's something so delightful about sharing with someone else the things you got on a successful shopping trip. Do you have someone with whom you can play "fashion show"? A girlfriend, your buddy, a sister, mother, husband, boyfriend, your kids? Share your success with a trusted person who will be happy for you. And if that isn't possible for some reason, then get dressed up in one of your new outfits and go out to the convenience store, coffee shop or a bookstore where you can parade through an aisle or two or around a few tables and check out who's checking you out! Feel as pretty as a peacock. Spread your beautiful feathers. You look great!

Fit in Fashion

Wow, what a shopping workout you've had! The effort you put into this is going to pay you back in so many ways. I hope you're celebrating. Just like any new sport you take on, it gets easier as you practice.

This is one of many successful shopping trips that you'll have. The warm-up exercises, the strategies you put into practice, the care you took to pace yourself will mean that next time it'll be easier, and easier again after that. So pat yourself on the back. You're doing great! As soon as possible, plan a date for your mixing and matching closet session. This is when you blend your new clothes with your old ones, put new outfits together and match those outfits to your style words.
Put a call into your buddy and ask her to join you.

Delightful things happen in this next session. And since you've been through the process of putting outfits together after you cleaned out your closet, you know what the steps are. Only now, your old clothes have new playmates to play off of and boy are you going to have fun! All sorts of surprises can show up. So don't delay.

Make that date with yourself!

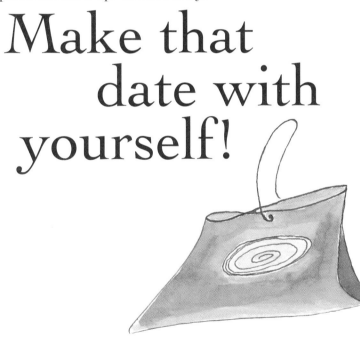

Completion and Renewal

I CAN SEE YOU NOW. You dashed home from your shopping trip and couldn't wait to tear into those packages to see if that lace top you bought would go with your brown twill pants. Or you're just waking up from a long rest after your shopping trip and only now are you curious about what's in those bags anyway. It may be a bit of a blur after your hunting expedition, but clarity is on its way.

One way or the other, you've arrived at this step where you let your new clothes meet and greet your older ones. This is such a fun part! After they check each other out, you'll probably notice some mating going on. Your newly purchased paisley shawl will snuggle against your two-year-old velvet skirt and fall instantly in love! Your ruffled skirt can't thank you enough for finding the open-toed sandals that will mean it gets to leave the closet and find its way onto the dance floor. Your twelve pairs of **pants finally have some tops to go with them** and they are so happy! You're the matchmaker and out-fits are going to leap out of that closet and bring you with them to all sorts of events. Not just work. Not just soccer games. Not just meet-ings. Those clothes have lots of living planned for you.

Matchmaking in the Closet

Have you put a call in for your buddy yet? Give her a ring and let her help celebrate your successful shopping day. Or, if it's midnight and you're revved up about your wardrobe, you can start without her. Pull out your **Wardrobe Workout Charts,** your portable rack if you have one, and your full-length mirror. Pull out your accessories as we did before, slip on a CD, crank the volume up and have some fun. You probably "finished" a lot of outfits by filling in the missing items on your shopping trip so go ahead and try those on. If it works the way you imagined it would, holler "Yippee!" and fill in the boxes in your

Wardrobe Workout Chart. If the outfit didn't come together as you expected, then see if you can figure out what would work instead. We plan ahead as best we can, but it doesn't always work out right. So if you realize an outfit would look better with a pointy-toed black boot instead of the square-toed one you bought (the pointy toed one is more racy), then make a note of the new, improved idea on a new shopping list, box up the boot you bought and plan to take it back this week.

Another thing that happens in this mixing/creating session is that MORE possibilities show up than you ever imagined. You weren't even looking for a top for your charcoal pants but the one you bought for your red corduroys looks FABULOUS with them. The sweater you bought to complete a dressy outfit might cross over and work miraculously with your jeans. Be open to many delightful surprises. This is like walking into a high school gym full of available men when you haven't had a date in months. There's a lot more to choose from now. More possibilities for getting it right.

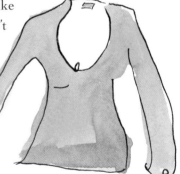

If you bought some more bottoms, pull out some blank **Wardrobe Workout Charts** and start charting the new outfits. You maximize your investment when you take the time to put the outfits together. It's great to be a good shopper, but until those clothes get together with each other and go out and play, your job isn't done. Team them up so you can forget about getting dressed and have more fun.

Remember, creative time is messy time! Expect your room to look as though a wild party has taken place. You might put your buddy to work keeping a little order in there so nothing gets buried. Or, ask her to work with the To Do list. You probably have some alterations to handle with your new clothes. Hems need taking up in pants or sleeve jackets need adjusting. Keep focused. Write things down that require action and make a plan for when you'll have that action completed.

Remember when I said that you'd make final decisions at home? You've probably already made some observations. Your purchases are either eagerly playing with lots of your clothes or they're standing off at the edge of your portable rack and not mixing in at all. Something you bought and expected would work one way might work twelve ways and something you were just sure would be great may not match up with your style words. If you were going for an edgier look, maybe the scarf you bought wasn't edgy enough. Keep telling the truth. Be completely satisfied. So what if this takes another shopping trip or two to get it right! You're going to be wearing these clothes for months or years so get it right right from the start. With practice you experience a lot more ease putting outfits together. This should make it much easier to give up something that you liked in the dressing room but doesn't work at home. There will always be more great things to shop for, and letting go of something that isn't working is easier when you understand this. It's easier to hunt and gather, harder to let go, so make a commitment only to those things that really work, that you just love and can't wait to wear.

Tweaking Your Wardrobe

It's not uncommon to have a few more things to buy even if you were conscientious and thorough your first shopping trip out. There will be some fine-tuning to do. Look for the details, like socks, hose and proper underwear to complete outfits. Fine tuning requires fine attention to detail. If you need a certain kind of black shoe to go with a particular dress, bring the dress with you on your next shopping trip. You'll most likely have fewer things on this "tweaking shopping list", but the attention you need to give them may be greater. Go for what works!

IT'S GOOD TO LET GO
When you get a crisp new white top to replace the old one, let the old one go.

While you put outfits together, you may also **weed things out.** Did you buy black pants that will replace the faded ones from last year? Let go of the items you successfully replaced. Now that you have a new crisp white top, get rid of the old limp one.

Put your buddy on "label control." Watch for tags that itch, show through a sheer fabric, or flip on the outside of your clothes. And take those labels off of the scarves too. No tags should distract the viewer from enjoying the beautiful portrait that is you.

If this means you're cutting out the care instructions, that's okay, because you're going to either staple those instructions to a note card with a description of the garment it came from or you'll attach them to a sheet of paper you keep near your laundry area. If you end up with a page full of care instructions, photocopy and laminate it for about a dollar. Keep it as a quick reference where you keep your laundry supplies.

Also, unless you already have a button jar going, put any extra buttons or beads that came with the garment in a zippered pouch that has three-ring punches and put it right in your binder. Keep like things together so you remember where they are and can find them when you need them.

Often it's when you have the new clothes at home and are putting things together that you pay more attention to the care instructions. If you realize that everything you bought needs to be dry cleaned, you may want to reconsider your buys at this time. Remember, if those clothes are constantly at the dry cleaners, you have to continue investing in them. If that's not a problem for you, fine. If it is, this is the right time to discover it — before you rip the tags off.

Once you've filled out your **Wardrobe Workout Charts** and put them in your binder, hung everything back on the hangers and slipped your clothes into your closet in color order, tucked your accessories away in their tidy spaces, made a pile of returns (if you have them) and put your receipts in your wallet or the bags or your binder so you have easy access to them, it's time to CELEBRATE! You've taken care of your wardrobe so it can take care of you. What better way to celebrate than to wear your clothes!

Wear Your Clothes

Now go out there and wear your clothes and don't save any of them for good. Remember, good is right now. Get used to it. Ordinary life is going to feel like a party. Wear your clothes for two weeks and listen for the compliments coming in. They may not be what you thought. You might hear things like:

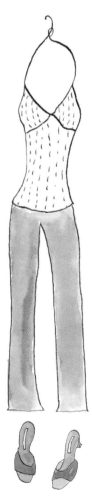

Have you been on vacation?

Is there a new love in your life?

Have you lost weight?

You look so radiant.

Are you pregnant?

What they may be thinking but aren't saying to your face is, "Have you had some surgery?" You will look markedly different, more different than a new outfit. So don't expect someone to say, "Hey, great outfit!" No, it'll look more like a transformation has happened. They'll imagine its much bigger than clothes.

So, how do you answer? You can make up anything you like when it comes to vacations or lovers. But you can keep it real simple if you like. In fact, I recommend it. When they say, "Gee you look great!", simply reply, **"Thank you."** No further explanation is necessary. Just graciously accept the compliment and move onto the next thing.

With your wardrobe together, you can go out and do other things like sign up for a class, start a hobby, take a trip, fall in love — and chances are, you have the clothes for it! And the time for it. You aren't spending any time worrying about your clothes and you're not fretting about not being able to find anything in your closet because it's all neat and tidy. You aren't saying, "I have NOTHING to wear!" because you have so many things to wear. Those problems are over. Kaput. Missing from your life.

There is **one little tiny thing** however. Remember when we started this project, I asked you to work with one season at a time? After the weeks and months go by, you will face that "other" season of clothes that are right now packed away somewhere. When it's time to do that, come back and take the quick system refresher course. In the meantime, take a look at these tips.

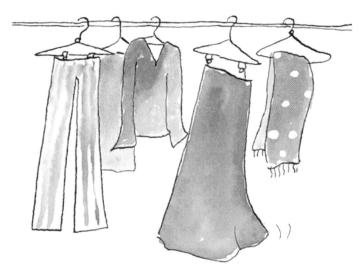

TIPS FOR STAYING CURRENT:

Things that need to be reviewed each season are makeup, hair, and eyewear.

MAKEUP: It's a great idea to schedule an appointment with a professional makeup artist and learn what new colors are out that are good for you this season. Generally you want to lighten up your makeup for summer and darken it for winter, adding drama around the holidays.

HAIR: Haircut alert! If your hair looks like it did three years ago or five years ago or ten years ago, you need an update. Get a new cut. That might mean going to a new hairdresser. "People-watch" for haircuts you like and ask them who does their hair.

Any processes applied to your hair really affect how your clothes look on you. If you are coloring, perming, or straightening your hair and you didn't do those things last year, then you need to take a closer look at your clothes and experiment more in dressing rooms, trying on different styles or fabrics. Generally, smooth hair likes smooth fabrics. Highly textured or patterned hair likes more texture and pattern.

BUY PRODUCTS: They're cheap. New technology is being developed all the time to help you have great hair and skin. Have faith. Throw out the half-used bottles under your bathroom sink. Technology has changed. Your skin and hair have changed. Catch up with yourself. If you bought a hair product and aren't getting the desired result, bring it back to your hair stylist and have him or her show you how to use it.

UPDATE YOUR COLORS: If your hair has changed colors or your skin has changed, chances are you should be wearing other colors. See a professional color analyst to help you make the right color choices for yourself in clothes and in makeup.

EYEWEAR: I realize that prescription glasses are expensive, but I have to insist that you take a look every year or two at the glasses you are wearing. Your glasses are your most important accessory so they need to be right. Because technology is advancing so quickly in this area, the trends in glasses change quickly too. Don't look outdated in your frames. Is this the year that you schedule an appointment to get new ones?

New Season System Refresher

After you've been wearing your outfits for a few months, the seasons will change. And that's when you'll go through this cycle pretty much as you did the first time. You may not spend as much time in Attitude Rehab because you've been practicing for several months already. But you'll still need to update. Each season is different and you're different in each season. You are living, breathing, changing, evolving, expanding, experimenting, exploring, and reaping the rewards of growing in your life. That's why you'll continue to show up for yourself and your clothes. I'll show you how.

Everything works better when it's maintained. Cars, teeth, and wardrobes all stay in better shape when you give them regular attention. Schedule an appointment with yourself for a style and wardrobe tune-up.

Next Steps for Each New Season

Here are some things to think about at the beginning of each season.

FILL IN THE BLANKS:

The one thing I am going to add to my wardrobe immediately is:

_____

Colors I will experiment with this year are:

_____

Accessories I want to shop for this season are:

_____

Services I am going to avail myself of this year are:

_____

_____

Look for qualities you respond to in images and name them. Whimsy, sensuality, sweetness, efficiency . . . What do you see?

What to Do When You Face a New Season

STEP 1 **Take advantage of the thick fashion magazines that come out at the beginning of each season, tear through them and rip out pictures of things you love.** Put your trimmed pages in sleeve protectors in your binder. Dump out the pictures from last year that you don't enjoy anymore. Keep only the ones that make you go "Wow! I love it!" Do you see any trends you'd like to adopt this season?

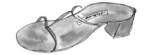

STEP 2 **Make a new collage, tack the images up on a bulletin board, or do something different.** Go to a card store and search for images that really resonate with you. Buy them. Take them home and analyze them as you would a dream. What are they trying to tell you? What is their essence? Is there some part of you that wants to be expressed? Look for qualities and name them, like whimsy, playfulness, sensuality, sassiness, sweetness, efficiency. If these words excite you, you're ready to "wear" them. Look at the Style Glossary for ideas on how to dress your new words. Are there other words in the Style Glossary that catch your attention? Try them on!

Write out your style recipe. If last season's style words fit for you, that's fine. Don't assume they will until you've done your collage work!

STEP 3 **Go through the interview questions again.** Have your needs changed? Have you moved? Has your job changed? Do you have more leisure time? Are you valuing your creativity and taking an art class? **Be open to even subtle changes.** Acknowledging subtle shifts can make a profound difference in the look you're going for now. Look out over the next few months. What's coming up? Weddings? Business trips? A reunion? A job change? Vacations? Add categories to your shopping list if they're new.

STEP 4 **Go back in the closet and pull out all the clothes you have for this season.** Try them on. For every item, ask these questions:

Does it fit? Is it flattering? Do I love it?

Weed out what's tattered, worn, unflattering, and unloved. Bring your buddy in to help you. Remember, silhouettes change. For five years clothes are oversized and boxy and then they take a turn and become form-fitting and lean. The transition from one year to the next can be subtle until the time comes when you try a jacket on and the silhouette is glaringly wrong on you. You haven't changed. Fashion has. Let go. It served you well.

STEP 5 **Look at your accessories.** Do you have shoes and handbags that look a little beat up? Take them to the shoe repair and have them revived. Pull out this season's jewelry. Does anything need repair?

STEP 6 **Downgrade some old favorites.** If you have some things that are looking a little shabby but you still love them to pieces, downgrade them. Instead of wearing last year's pants for dressy events this year, wear them for casual. Instead of wearing the long flowy garden dress as a dress, downgrade it to a nightgown. Instead of wearing your ankle pants for your casual work setting, downgrade their moderately worn selves to serve as yoga pants instead. You'll still get lots of pleasure from these older models, but just in different parts of your life.

STEP 7 **Follow the same rules for cleaning your closet as you did in Closet Resolve.** Pull out anything that grew in there that isn't related to clothing. Weeding out the rubble, putting your clothes back in color order, and adding a nice smelling sachet to a couple of hangers will do a lot for getting you into the spirit of the season. It feels so good! Do it for that reason alone. Open those closet doors and see order, cleanliness, and ease. You deserve this kind of peace in a closet all year long.

Go back now and read the Fashion Quiz and Wardrobe Bill of Rights in Chapter One. Sit quietly for a few minutes and reflect on how it used to be.

STEP 8 **Take inventory again.** Did anything get terribly out of balance? Too many party clothes and not enough work clothes? Still no solution to your date wardrobe? Work at finding the difficulty and focus your attention on that area first.

STEP 9 **Create your shopping list.** Get out your Wardrobe Workout Charts and start making new outfits. Start as early in the season as you can to shop for what you need. Some things really do fly off the shelves. I don't want you going in on December 12th looking for long silk underwear and not finding it because it all sold out a month ago.

STEP 10 **Once you have shopped for the new things on your list, go home and do the mixing-and-matching dance with your clothes, staying up till all hours, happily charting the outfits (on your Wardrobe Workout Charts) you'll be wearing over the next few months.** Put your notes in your binder. And then go out and wear your clothes! Your system has been upgraded and refreshed.

Once you've been through each season, you're back at the anniversary of when you started this process. Now you can align yourself with nature to help keep your momentum. Does the term "spring cleaning" mean anything to you? It could be called "fall cleaning" as well. There's a natural wardrobe rhythm in the few weeks between winter and spring and summer and fall when invisible fashion fairies flutter near your shoulders and nudge you toward your closet. It's a great feng shui thing to do regularly, too — organize, de-clutter, put order into your closet. According to that ancient Chinese practice of right placement, the rest of your life will work better, too.

Look How Far You've Come

So, how are you doing? How satisfied are you? Sometimes we are so ready for change that when the steps show up and we take them, we can hardly remember where we were when we started. I invite you to revisit that now. Go back and do the fashion quiz in chapter one. Compare your answers now to when we first started working together. Most likely, you had quite a few yeses back then. Do you have considerably more nos this time? Look at the Wardrobe Bill of Rights again. When you read each statement attach a percentage to it that correlates to how much that statement lives inside as your truth. Are you closer to feeling the truth of those statements 100 percent of the time?

Sit quietly for a few minutes reflecting on how it used to be and how it is now. Would you say you are wildly satisfied with your results or mildly satisfied? If you're **wildly satisfied**, great! You did the work, you are getting the results. You've learned some new habits, you're on track!

If you're mildly satisfied, let's do some troubleshooting and see where we can go to improve your results.

How did the buddy system work for you? If you went through the workbook without a buddy, maybe it's time you got one. They really can escalate your growth. If you had a buddy, maybe you need a different one. Or, how about getting a buddy team? I have a few teams in my life and I wouldn't be half as successful as I am without them. Buddies really do help you get the job done.

Or, if a buddy isn't your thing, consider calling a professional image consultant to help you. A great resource is the Association of Image Consultants International (1-972/755-1503) or go to their web site: www.aici.org. for a referral in your area.

If going through Attitude Rehab was particularly tough, maybe you have some deeper issues that could use some professional help. Ask your friends or at church for some therapy referrals. Often the issues of self-esteem and self-worth which come up around clothes can be handled effectively in a therapeutic setting. You're worth it! Get more help!

If shopping wasn't very successful for you, hold tight. It just may not be your season. Sometimes your style and what's out there aren't a perfect match. But, there's always next season! If you'd like some ideas of what to do in the meantime, check out the chapter "What To Do When Current Fashion Sucks" in *40 Over 40: 40 Things Every Woman Over 40 Needs to Know About Getting Dressed*.

If you're prioritizing and doing your shopping more slowly — filling in what you need a bit at a time — it'll take a little longer to have the full results. Be patient. Each day that you're wearing only what you love, even if that means there are only three things to choose from, you're doing great. Just keep adding things you love when you can. And don't be surprised if someone shows up with a few things they were letting go of and they thought of you and gee, they just happen to be perfect. That's how grace works. Once you're clear, things happen. If you keep focused on the exercises we did, your wardrobe will show up sooner than you think.

Go back to the Tell-the-truth-Let-go-Create mantra. Are you pausing long enough in your busy life to really hear yourself tell the truth about what you love, need and want? Keep staying current with your insides. You have to know what's going on there before you can dress the

Let go of the past. Let go of mistakes or bad choices and look forward to the next opportunity to get it right.

outsides. So if you skipped over the exercises or the collage work, you know right where you need to go. Go back and do those exercises!

There are lots of tools in this workbook. Fall back into these pages and find the ones that will help you through when you hit the bumps in the road. If illness befalls you, you will shore yourself up with your clothes, knowing that looking good will help you feel good. If your relationship goes under, your clothes will help you recover your sense of self so you can go back out there and stand tall and proud even if you still hurt inside. Keep my voice in your ear. Clothes comfort, heal, revive, and renew. Let them be that for you.

Stay current. Let go of the past, even if the past is as recent as last week. Let go of mistakes or bad choices and look forward to the next opportunity to get it right. Live with what you love. Let love be all there is.

When you come across a rut, be happy you saw it. Now you have the tools to get out of it. Keep pulling pictures to guide you. Keep people - watching for new ideas. Keep practicing the fashion strategies. You'll have lots of opportunities to forget what you've learned, to lose your way. That's okay. It happens to all of us. Even me. We're human, remember? All I expect is that you **keep practicing** being kind and loving to yourself. I want you satisfied.

Time to Celebrate!

May I just add something here? Look where you are! And just think back to when you first held this book in your hand. Remember where you were then? Feeling a little (or a lot) hopeless, helpless, desperate, unsatisfied. Now look at yourself! You kept your commitment. You faced your wardrobe demons and bad programming. You made it through Attitude Rehab and have successfully practiced your fashion strategies. You stopped being so hard on yourself. You found solutions in places where you didn't expect them.

And you didn't do this alone. You surrounded yourself with people who had good vibes, people who supported you — and you stayed away from the ones who didn't. You got a buddy or you became a buddy to yourself.

You did your homework. You made your collages and listened to their wisdom. You went through the interview questions and gained

You may have shed a tear or two, talked over your clothing issues with someone else, got some freedom — and now look at you! Free to forget about your looks and go out there and live your divine life.

clarity. You figured out who you are right now and made the connection between your clothes and yourself.

You did the grunt work in your closet, moved out the old, brought in the new. You may have shed a tear or two, talked over your clothing issues with someone else, got some freedom, moved past the hard memories, celebrated your accomplishments — and now look at you! After some clearing, sorting, shopping, and some sessions of putting outfits together, you are expressing YOURSELF in clothes. **You are so perfectly YOU!** Free to forget about your looks and go out there and live your divine life.

It's time to celebrate. I can imagine you and your girlfriends — your buddy and other buddies — going out for a fun night together, enjoying each other, complimenting each other and talking about all that you have been through. It's great to see a project to completion and celebrating is the last step.

Your Testimonial

If you've gone through the steps in this book, then it's very likely you've experienced a transformation — or maybe two or three or twenty. You might be interested to hear what other women have said who, like you, have created a wardrobe from the inside out. Here are their testimonials:

"This has shown me how much I know about what I really like. It's helpful to understand my own intuition and trust myself."

"I feel like the 'me' that was forgotten."

"I get so many compliments."

"I gave myself permission to be myself and now I feel so much stronger and more confident."

"Colleagues are responding so differently to me. I'm showing my self-respect through the way I dress."

*"This has really simplified my life.
It's not a vanity thing.
It feels so right being put together."*

"I never would have believed shopping could be fun."

"I really can look like someone who will be taken seriously. I really accomplished what I wanted - being able to look powerful and beautiful at the same time."

*"I've made a very positive career change.
They recruited me largely based on my
professional and upscale image."*

*"Clothes are so personal, and I wasn't taking
them personally until now. Now I am and it
makes me so happy."*

What's your testimonial? Share it with your buddy and share it with me at
bkinsel@brendakinsel.com

WRITE IT NOW:

_____

_____

_____

_____

_____

When I hear how a transformed wardrobe has transformed a woman's life, I no longer question the value, importance, and power in the simple act of getting dressed.

Just Remember

You've invested thought, time, energy and money into your wardrobe. Make that investment work for you every single day. When you've outgrown your look, do your homework and find the new one — the one that reflects the current you. Remember, everything that looks effortless has effort behind it. When you take the steps to work through your wardrobe, it will support you by being effortless. Take time for yourself. You're worth it.

We are all going to be facing things in our lives. Job opportunities, new babies, love interests, praise for good service to the community. And there will be tough times, too, and losses, when your confidence and well-being are as challenged as a major league baseball team during the playoffs. My wish is that you'll have faith and friends to help you in those times, but I also hope you'll remember where you've tucked support away for yourself. Inside your closet, your clothes are there for you — to comfort you, to help you feel good, to celebrate with you, to enhance your life and make you look good. Remember, when you look good, you feel good.

Share what you have learned with others And do it the buddy way — with kindness.

Spread the Love

Remember from historical accounts how Native Americans would use every part of the animal they killed? A buffalo supplied food, shelter, clothing, soap, tools, jewelry, and more. Every part of that animal was used. Nothing was wasted.

You started this book with some idea of what you wanted. I imagine more things have been accomplished than you thought. Now **I challenge you** to take this book apart and use it in all aspects of your life. You could take the same steps you used to clean out your closet and tackle your pantry, bookshelves, linen closet, catch-all drawer, kitchen cupboards, you name it — and eliminate all that's not necessary so what's necessary (and loved) can have more prominence in your life. Bring beauty and order into other areas of your home.

Take the interview questions and apply them to your personal or business life. The Moving Away From, Moving Toward Exercise can be applied to your family life, relationships, career or your spirituality, and it can yield clarity, insight, and direction for you. Are you at a crossroads in your life? Do the On Becoming Exercise or the I Need ____ , I Want ____ Exercise. Look at your work life and do the I Used to ____ , but Now I ____ Exercise and see how you want to expand and grow. Do it with your finances in mind. These are great all-purpose tools that can be applied to anything. Use them.

The most effective way to learn something is to teach it. Take the fashion strategies and teach them wherever you can. **Share them** with children and young adults. Help them get off to a good start by accepting themselves as they are, enjoying their bodies, discovering what they love, and having fun with clothes. Give them that freedom. Share this good sense with your sister, your niece, your friends, your mom. *Spread the love.* Champion the rights of women to be happy and whole, strong and confident, and encourage them to demonstrate that every day through their second skin, their clothes. Clothes are our closest and strongest form of expression. Bathe yourself in that expression and help others do the same, but not in a big sister bossy way. Do it in the buddy way — with kindness.

Be well. Be joyous. Be free and have fun. When you have a problem and you don't know what to do, go tidy up your closet. The answers will come. Be kind. In small ways each day, build your bank account of appreciation. Then get up tomorrow and do it again. In the words of the Navajo Prayer, spread the love.

Love before me
Love behind me
Love to the right of me
Love to the left of me
Love above me
Love below me
Love within me
Love all around me.

I think of you always. Enjoy this splendid journey discovering and rediscovering your true nature. We are so blessed to have each other and to have these miraculous bodies to clothe and care for. Get up, get dressed, and get out there.

I can't wait to see you!

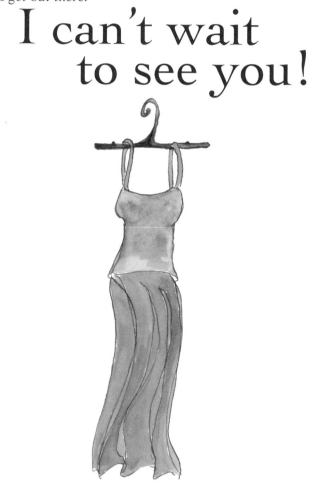

About the Author

BRENDA KINSEL is the owner of Inside Out, A Style and Wardrobe Consulting Company, founded in 1985. She matches clothes to the personalities, lifestyles and passions of her clients through her continuing consulting work.

Her first book, the best-selling *40 over 40: 40 Things Every Woman Over 40 Needs to Know About Getting Dressed*, was a finalist in the category of women's issues for the Independent Publisher's Book Awards (the IPPYS) in 2001. She is also the author of *In the Dressing Room with Brenda: A Fun and Practical Guide to Buying Smart and Looking Great.* Her books are translated into several languages.

She is also the fashion editor for the *Pacific Sun* newspaper, where she's been writing a monthly column since 1995. Her advice and expertise have been showcased on television shows including The Oprah Winfrey Show, Men are from Mars, Women are from Venus, Fox News, and in the pages of national magazines including *InStyle, Shape, Weight Watchers*, and internationally in   a leading Swedish magazine for women over forty. She's also been featured in many newspapers including the *Chicago Tribune, the Boston Globe, the Detroit Free Press, the San Jose Mercury News* and others. She is, as well, a regular on the popular Jack and Sandy Show on KFGO radio in Fargo, North Dakota.

As a speaker on fashion and women's issues, Brenda entertains standing room only crowds in retail stores that include Macy's, Marshall Field's, Nordstrom, and smaller boutiques nationwide. She also speaks to professional organizations and associations.

She is a past president of the San Francisco Bay Area Chapter of the Association of Image Consultants International (AICI) and served fours years on AICI's international board. She received AICI's most prestigious award, the IMMIE (Image Makers Merit of Industry Excellence), in 2000 for achievement in the image industry.

Brenda grew up on a farm in southeastern North Dakota near a town called Hastings, population 75, where all the women were great dressers. She is the proud mother of three wonderful adult kids, Caitlin, Erin, and Trevor, who have a knack for looking great. She lives in Marin County, California.

For further information about Brenda's services and appearances,
or to view her monthly newsletter, Tips & Teasers,
visit her online at www.brendakinsel.com.
You can also e-mail her at bkinsel@brendakinsel.com
or write to her at PO Box 657, Ross, CA 94957

About the Illustrator

JENNY PHILLIPS has been a graphic designer for sixteen years. Her work ranges from launching new products to designing identities and creating whimsical illustrations about popular culture. She is the principal of JuMP Studio in San Francisco. The studio provides art direction, marketing communications, graphic design services and illustrations for a wide variety of commercial and not-for-profit organizations.

About the Press

WILDCAT CANYON PRESS publishes books that embrace such subjects as friendship, spirituality, women's issues, and home and family, all with a focus on self-help and personal growth. Great care is taken to create books that inspire reflection and improve the quality of our lives. Our books invite sharing and are frequently given as gifts.

For a catalog of our publications
Please write:
Wildcat Canyon Press
Council Oak Books
1615 S Baltimore, Suite 3
Tulsa, OK 74119
Phone (918) 587-6454
Fax (918) 583-4995
www.wildcatcanyon.com
www.counciloakbooks.com

Other Books by Brenda Kinsel

40 over 40:
40 Things Every Woman Over 40 Needs to Know About Getting Dressed
Brenda Kinsel with illustrations by Jenny M. Phillips
Wildcat Canyon $16.95 / $26.25 Canada, Trade paperback, ISBN 1-885171-42-0, 192 pages, 6 X 8, 24 original illustrations, Two-color throughout

It's tough to be a woman over forty in a world where fashion is dominated by youth and unattainable body images. But help is on the way! With generous doses of humor, 40 over 40 speaks to the woman who is forty or over, helping her develop style and expression through her clothes. It provides a compassionate voice to the busy woman who has been befuddled by fashion maybe forever, and now that she perceives she is over the "fashion hill," she's really lost. While acknowledging the changes she's gone through in the past decades, 40 over 40 takes her through the steps that will make getting dressed an extraordinarily satisfying experience. It dissects the fashion and beauty business, pulls out what works, and shows the reader how to toss out what doesn't. This stylish and sassy book delivers straight talk to the woman over forty, helping her appear every bit as successful and accomplished on the outside as she is on the inside.

In the Dressing Room with Brenda:
A Fun and Practical Guide to Buying Smart and Looking Great
Brenda Kinsel with illustrations by Jenny M. Phillips
$16.95 / $26.25 Canada, Trade paperback, ISBN 1-885171-51-X, 224 pages, 6 x 8, Color illustrations

Personal shopping advice from every woman's favorite image consultant, Brenda Kinsel. Famous for talking about things that people think about but don't always say out loud, Brenda Kinsel tackles underwear, the booty, and the nightmare of shopping with kids (please pass the Valium!) — all while helping women make sense out of the vast imponderable that is the world of fashion. With gentle understanding, she helps every woman develop a healthier relationship with herself by taking a lighter look at hang-ups, and a deeper look at the fashion traps that are out there ready to grab the unsuspecting consumer.

NOTES:

NOTES:

NOTES:

NOTES:

NOTES:

NOTES:

NOTES: